The Veterinary Sup...

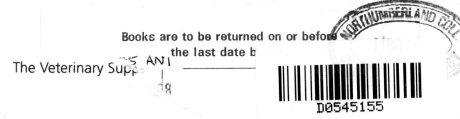

D0545155

From the re

What a pity this book was not written before I became a
practice manager! ...an easy-to-read style. Maggie Shilcock's
book... is a must for practice libraries and for those considering
joining a veterinary practice.   Penny Bredemear **VN Times**

...this book is a starting point for providing the veterinary
support team with the training tools that they need. ...for new
entrants into and the progressing members of the veterinary
support team.
        Christine Ann Merle DVM MB **editorial@penguin.doody.com**

Pocket Practice Guides

Series Editors: Carl Gorman BVSc MRCVS and Sue Gorman BVSc MRCVS

Clients, Pets and Vets:
Communication and management
Carl Gorman

Finance, Employment and Wealth for Vets
Second Edition
Keith Dickinson

The Veterinary Support Team
Maggie Shilcock

Premises for Vets
Designing the Veterinary Habitat
Jim Wishart

Interviewing and Recruiting Veterinary Staff
Maggie Shilcock

Pocket Practice Guides

The Veterinary Support Team

Maggie Shilcock
BSc CMS

Illustrated by Hayley Albrecht

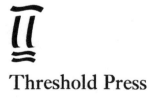

Threshold Press

First published in 2001 by
Threshold Press Ltd, 152 Craven Road, Newbury
Berks RG14 5NR
Phone 01635-528375 and fax 01635-36294
email: publish@threshold-press.co.uk
www.threshold-press.co.uk

Reprinted 2001, 2002

ISBN 1–903152–06–2

Available in USA and Canada from
Iowa State University Press
A Blackwell Science Company
2121 S. State Avenue
Ames, IA 50014-8300
(Orders Tel: 800-862-6657, Fax: 515-292-3349
 Web: www.isupress.com, email: orders@isupress.com)

Designed by Jim Weaver Design
Typeset by Threshold Press Ltd
Printed in England by Biddles Ltd, Guildford and Kings Lynn

The Illustrator
Hayley Albrecht obtained an honours degree in silversmithing at
Loughborough in 1996 and has worked in this field and as an artist
ever since. Since the last Pocket Practice Guide she has started
exhibiting in London, and was an award winner at the Society of
Equestrian Artists annual exhibition at Christies in 2000.
Although accompanied and inspired by her remaining animals, the
pictures in this book are dedicated to Tammy the dog, who spent
patient hours sleeping under the drawing board while they were
being created, and whose presence will be sadly missed.

Contents

Preface

Ask any non-pet owner of the late twentieth century (and yes there are a few, despite the veterinary docusoaps) to paint you a picture of a veterinary practice and, like as not, they will describe for you a cosy, 1930s Herriotesque scene with wooden furniture and a homely lady who answers the phone when not doing the dusting.

Ask the same question of a 21st century pet owner and they will draw a picture of the modern, efficient, technologically up-to-date specialist small animal practice that is to be found, now not only in our cities, but throughout the land. Small animal practice is the success story of the late 20th century but it takes a veterinary sociologist to point out the impact of these differences on the people who work in the practices. Just as there has been and explosion in small animal expertise and facilities, so the has been a parallel one in the number and skills of staff needed to support it, both clinically and non-clinically. Whilst the science has fuelled the expansion in expertise, it is the people who have fashioned its image and culture.

It was the foresight of a few pioneers in the 60s and 70s who realised that their clients, the pet owners, were becoming a more and more sophisticated group of consumers, and that good medicine alone was not going to be enough to ensure success in an ever more competitive world. They brought us practice management as a vital addition to the 'hands on' practicality of the Herriot era. With better management has come a divide-and-conquer approach. With vets vetting and nurses nursing, a raft of skilled employees has developed to cover the myriad of reception, financial, legal and IT skills required to operate a practice. Many practices now employ between six and eight support staff per vet.

This volume, covering as it does the whole range of skills required by this team, serves to highlight how totally dependant those privileged to work with the letters MRCVS after their names are on this loyal, dedicated, long suffering, and (dare we say it) often undervalued group of workers. Maggie Shilcock's long experience of hands-on practice management has produced a review of the whole field that will be useful to new entrant and progressing staff members alike, and it won't come amiss to a few partners to remind themselves just how much their support staff do. It is interesting to reflect that in recent discussions for the Veterinary Practice

Management Association's Veterinary Practice Administration Certificate, colleges refused to believe that any employers could ask their staff to be competent at so many tasks!

There is little doubt that we ask our staff to enter a more stressful environment than existed in veterinary practice of late. Stress management seems to have become as important a skill as financial expertise for today's practice manager, but stress is mostly feeling loss of control, and control comes from more knowledge. A mastery of the subjects contained within these covers will surely lead to a skilled, successful, and above all, happy progression through a veterinary practice career.

Roger Haverson B.Vet.Med. MRCVS
Chairman, Education Committee VPMA
February 2001

Acknowledgements

My grateful thanks go to the support staff at The Veterinary Hospital, Estover Plymouth, Devon; Bishopton Veterinary Group, Ripon, North Yorkshire and Heacham and Priory Court Veterinary Clinics, at Heacham and South Wootton, Norfolk, for their help in compiling the 'What support staff say' sections at the end of each chapter.

Thanks also to Roger my partner for his support and advice and for providing me with a sounding board when writing this book.

1

Support staff – so who are they and what do they do?

I have always wanted to work in a veterinary surgery
I have always loved animals, I have four dogs, three cats, a rabbit and
four hamsters at home.

These are two of the commonest reasons given by job applicants for support staff vacancies in veterinary practice. There's much more to this job however than loving animals.

Working in a veterinary practice is still seen as glamorous, it has a certain romance about it, all the more enhanced by the numerous TV programmes about veterinary practices. After all, support staff are directly or indirectly involved in saving the lives of little and large furry creatures. The 'ah' factor also plays an important part in wanting to work at the vet's. None of us can deny it – who hasn't moved around the reception counter to stroke the new puppy or kitten, brought in for its first vaccination. If a receptionist or nurse didn't love animals, it would be a difficult job to do, the client may be causing them to tear their hair out but at least the dog or cat is pretty!

Many support staff are working in veterinary practice because they have a genuine need to help in the care of animals and see this type of job as in some measure achieving their ambition.

However, support staff cannot afford to be too sentimental, there are sad situations every day in veterinary practice, euthanasias, road traffic accidents, lost pets and homeless kittens brought in. The waifs and strays cannot all be taken home, or the treasured dog killed by the speeding car be replaced. Sadness – as well as joy – are all part of the daily routine in practice and support staff have to be able to cope. They need to be realistic but compassionate, sympathetic but not too sentimental and above all patient.

Sympathy is needed when an animal is euthanased, understanding is needed when a client's dog pees on the newly washed floor, assertiveness is needed when asking clients to pay and politeness is needed always, even with the most difficult of clients. It's a tall order.

Tall order it may be, but there are still lots of applicants when support staff jobs in veterinary practices are advertised. So what do support staff actually do, what skills do they need and what do clients expect of them, what qualities should they possess? In this chapter we are going to answer these questions as well as look at the many different 'hats' support staff have to wear each day.

Who are they?

Support staff are all the people working in veterinary practice who are not veterinary surgeons.

The function of support staff is to support the veterinary surgeons in the work they do, and enable the smooth and efficient running of the practice while the veterinary surgeons carry out their clinical role. It's the support staff who answer the telephone, book the appointments, deal with the difficult client, send out invoices, follow up bad debts, do practice accounts, organise rotas, the list is endless, and oh yes, it is also they who make the coffee and wash up all the dirty cups in the staff room!

The whole spectrum of practice support roles are carried out by these employees. Their jobs vary from full-time practice manager to the receptionist who may only work a few hours a week, as well as the non-clinical aspects of a veterinary nurse's role.

Let's look at some of these roles in more detail.

Receptionists

The receptionist is the 'front of house' staff member who is responsible for organising client appointments and answering client queries, either over the telephone or in the waiting room. The role does not, however, end there. She is also likely to be responsible for generating client bills and accounts and for debt control. Receptionists are key members of staff when it comes to promoting practice services, new veterinary products, nursing clinics and pet insurance. They are the practice's 'listening ear' and some of the most important public relations people in the practice. Many receptionists also dispense veterinary medicines and products, a role which requires knowledge as well as great care and attention to detail.

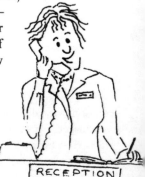

RECEPTION

Book-keepers

Book-keepers are often employed on a part-time basis to organise the practice accounts and VAT returns. They may also produce financial accounts for the practice manager or managing partner.

Secretaries

Many larger practices employ full or part-time secretarial staff who produce veterinary reports, deal with practice correspondence and who are often, because of their word processing skills, involved in the production of practice newsletters, leaflets and posters.

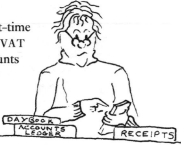

Administrative staff

Administrative staff may be responsible for dealing with client pet Insurance claims, organising RSPCA, PDSA and other animal charity work which the practice carries out. They may also help clients find charity funding to pay for their veterinary bills. Large animal practices often have a member of staff whose responsibility it is to log all farm visits onto the computer and to generate farmers' accounts and chase any bad debts.

Veterinary nurses

Both qualified and non-qualified veterinary nurses are involved in non-clinical roles in the veterinary practice. This may be as head nurse managing a team of nurses or organising rotas, a trainee nurse who has responsibility for filing clients' lab reports and x-rays or the nurse doing her stint on the reception desk.

What experience do you need?

Support staff come with a variety of experience and from many backgrounds, but the one thing they all have in common is a love of animals and a strong desire to work in a veterinary practice.

The vast majority of support staff who apply for non-nursing jobs in veterinary practice have had little or no previous experience of the veterinary environment. With the exception perhaps of owning their own pet and therefore using a veterinary surgery as a client, or having had a school work-experience placement in a veterinary practice. Of course it is an advantage if you have worked in a veterinary practice before, but this lack of experience has never really mattered especially as, in many cases, support staff have previously worked as receptionists in other service industries. Experience gained in dealing with the public will stand anyone in good stead for working in a veterinary practice, where dealing with animals is the least difficult of their tasks. Dealing with the public is often far harder! No-one should be deterred from applying for a support staff role in a veterinary practice just because they have no previous direct veterinary experience.

The road to veterinary nursing is somewhat different; many nurses are taken on as school leavers to be trained by the practice and then go on to take their two-year veterinary nursing qualification. Many trainee nurses will already have worked in the practice as volunteers, Saturday staff, or as work-experience students. For purely nursing jobs a practice will usually be looking for either trainee nurses or qualified and/or experienced nurses who have worked in practice and taken their veterinary nursing exams, or perhaps even nursing diplomas in a specialist area of veterinary nursing.

What age should you be?

There are opportunities for all age groups to join the veterinary support staff team, from mothers returning to part-time work to school and college leavers looking for a full-time career in veterinary practice.

What about formal education?

Much of an employee's day in a veterinary practice is spent communicating with clients and staff, face to face, on the telephone, fax or email, so the employee must be articulate. Knowing how to relate to people – people skills – are an absolute essential. Support staff must be good communicators both at work with staff and clients, and outside with Mrs. Bloggs in the supermarket, when she just has to stop them in the frozen food isle to tell them how much better or worse little Gemma her poodle is or, worse, to complain about her last vet's bill. People skills will be stretched to their limit in situations like this, but they must never snap.

An ability to write good English is essential, as well as being able to convey information clearly and concisely to and from clients, vets and staff. Numeracy is also vital, even though many practices now have computerised client accounts and there is no longer a need to add up the client's bill at the end of the consultation.

The need for computer skills goes without saying, although some practices still do not have computerised accounts or client databases.

More and more practices have email and websites and many produce their own in-house newsletters on PCs to a very high standard. All staff members need to have a sound basic knowledge of Microsoft Windows or equivalent and be able to adapt their computer knowledge to the particular veterinary software used by the practice.

Most practices look for support staff with a good basic education, often the equivalent of today's four or five GCSEs. Veterinary nurses currently require five GCSEs at grades C or above to be accepted on the RCVS/BVNA veterinary nurse training course and this is becoming a requirement even for those nurses who do not train to be VNs.

Equality of the sexes

There are very few male receptionists in veterinary practice but there are an increasing number of male employees in the more administrative and management roles.

Historically and currently veterinary support staff are not especially well paid and, as mentioned earlier, many are part-time. This does not appeal financially to men and goes some way to explaining why many support staff jobs are taken by older females returning to work to earn an extra income, but not a wage to support a family.

It is pleasing to find a small but increasing number of male veterinary nurses and to see Nick Taylor elected as the 2000 President of the BVNA. Hopefully this will encourage more men to enter the profession from school.

How should you look?

Well – smart, appropriately dressed, tidy, well groomed, these are some of the terms used as qualities which are looked for at interviews.

Jeans, trainers and a sweatshirt may be worn at home but at work it's different, what support staff wear and how they look must reflect the professional practice image. The practice must think of its clients; clients expect veterinary staff to be professionals and their appearance has to reflect this, a sloppily dressed vet, nurse or receptionist shouts out sloppy work, and no client wants that for their pets. Many practices provide uniforms and/or have a dress code which employees must follow, including quite often the banning of all jewellery except wedding rings.

Being a team member

Support staff have to be team members – able to work alongside other staff and vets in the practice. They will probably be part of a small specialist team such as receptionists or nurses, as well as being a member of the whole practice team. This means working together to achieve results, not going off to 'do their own thing' because they think they can do it better. They also have to be committed to the practice. It's part of the culture of veterinary practice that the job ends when the last animal goes home. They may be working long hours, or extra hours if there is an emergency – it's all part of the job.

They have to be flexible, able to stay that extra half-hour while the last minute appointment is seen, even if it is only a booster, which could easily have been seen tomorrow. And they have to be cheerful about it – no room here for moaning Minnies!

Jack and Jill of all trades

Working in a veterinary practice is not a soft option, support staff work can be hard, involving long hours and stretched emotions. One of the characteristics of veterinary practices is that many jobs are multi-roled. Support staff need to be able to juggle a number of jobs – book Mrs Black's appointment, while remembering to return her cat's booster vaccination record once the vet has signed it, pass Mrs. Brown's dog's urine sample to the lab, while remembering to phone Mrs. Green about collecting her cat's tablets, oh, and not forgetting to change the poster display in the waiting room, restock the dog food stand and finally print out the information the vet requested from the computer. And that's just before coffee!

Many practices employ support staff who act as nurse/receptionists, these staff help the veterinary surgeons in the consulting room and the theatre as well as acting as receptionists. Other practices employ dedicated receptionists and nurses who concentrate on their own specialist roles within the practice

The variety of different jobs support staff undertake can be awe-inspiring, but if you ask any member of a veterinary practice what they like most about their job, they will almost certainly answer, 'the variety, we never know what we may be doing from day to day, it's a great challenge'.

Figure 1 The Qualities of Veterinary Support Staff

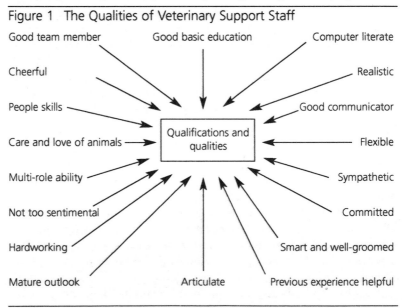

Good team member   Good basic education   Computer literate

Cheerful   Realistic

People skills   Good communicator

Care and love of animals ——→   Qualifications and   ←—— Flexible
                                 qualities

Multi-role ability   Sympathetic

Not too sentimental   Committed

Hardworking   Smart and well-groomed

Mature outlook   Articulate   Previous experience helpful

What do the clients think support staff do?

Probably not as much as we all imagine. Here is where there is a need for a bit of client education, which isn't just about pet health care.

Whether nurse or receptionist, it is important that clients appreciate support staff roles and skills. It is actually a relatively easy matter to explain the roles of the staff to clients by use of practice brochures, websites and displays.

Clients will be interested and surprised at the number of different responsibilities support staff have. Who do they think sends the boosters or accounts, updates records, fills in insurance forms, organises the lost and found notice board, arranges for RSPCA contributions towards clients bills and so on and so on?

Do clients know the training required to become a VN, and the kind of knowledge and skills they have once trained? Do they know what they do behind the scenes, how they care for pre- and post op. animals and the newborn, or help take x-rays?

If the clients think that receptionists just make appointments and collect the money, then the practice needs to be telling them otherwise. It's good public relations and clients love to know more about the workings of their veterinary practice and the people who work in it.

What do support staff really do?

However long a list of jobs a member of support staff may produce when asked what they do, I can guarantee that they will miss a significant number from their list.

These missing jobs are the secondary roles all members of support staff play in veterinary practice.

The straightforward primary roles of nurse, receptionist, dispenser, bookkeeper, and administrator will be dealt with later in the book. Here we are going to look at all the other secondary roles which are carried out every day without even knowing it.

Friend

This is probably the most important secondary role support staff carry out. They are the client's friends. It's the receptionist they phone for the appointment and then talk to for five minutes on the phone, listing every symptom their pet is exhibiting. It's the receptionist they see first in the waiting room and tell all their troubles to. It's often the receptionist they ask to explain again just how they give their pet its medication. as they can't quite remember what the vet said they had to do. It's the nurse who takes their animal away for its operation and explains what is going to happen, and it's the nurse who brings it back to them, drowsy but alive and

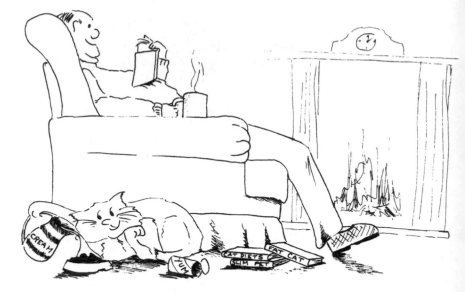

well and talks to them about how well the operation went. Support staff are the ones they tell that the diet given to Bonzo by the practice nurse is working wonderfully but 'he does like his biscuit last thing at night when I have my cup of Horlicks'.

Counsellor, comforter, social worker

Sometimes the role changes from that of friend to counsellor. The bereaved client, whose dog was their only companion, needs to talk to someone and often it's support staff who have to take on this role. The client whose cat has been in a road traffic accident (RTA) and who blames herself because she left the downstairs window open, often needs to talk to a receptionist about how guilty she feels. The receptionists can't change what has happened for these clients but they can listen.

Theirs may be the shoulder that is cried upon when the client's pet is euthanased or it may be their comforting words in this, or other sad situations which don't of course always involve the client's pet. The staff in a veterinary surgery are often perceived as people to whom troubles can be told, so they may find themselves hearing about a client's feud with their neighbour, a marriage break-up or, heaven forbid, the blow-by-blow account of their stay in hospital. Whatever the scenario they are providing a listening and confidential ear. There is of course a limit to the amount of time they can spend in this way, they do have other jobs to do and it is here that their tact and diplomacy must come into play. However, time spent listening to clients is a good investment for a practice and something the veterinary surgeon does not always have time for.

Diplomat

Support staff need to exercise their diplomacy both with clients and with staff. Receptionists don't tell clients why their favourite vet is in hospital or where he has gone on his holidays, even if the clients are on their hands and knees pleading for the information. And then there's the client who wants to discuss another client's case, or is criticising another local veterinary surgery or even another member of the practice staff. The receptionists have to listen but of course cannot comment, only try to steer the conversation in other directions.

Charity organiser

All veterinary practices have charity boxes in their waiting rooms to help raise funds for animals in distress, but the other side of the coin is the organising of help for clients who are having difficulty paying their bills. It is normally the support staff who are instrumental in liaising between organisations such as the RSPCA, NCDL, PDSA and the client, as well as dealing with the paperwork involved in such matters.

If the practice has open days it is likely to be raising money for at least one animal charity, so they will probably be helping to organise charity stands or maybe a raffle, the proceeds of which will go to the charity.

Debt collector

This doesn't sound very appealing, but it is what receptionists sometimes have to be, and usually they will be far more effective than any outside debt collecting agency because of their personal approach.

All veterinary practices have some bad debtors and it tends to be the receptionist who has the responsibility for calling in the overdue account either by repeated letters or telephone calls. Even more difficult is persuading the reluctant client to hand over the money, or come back later in the day with the cash they have conveniently left at home. Some receptionists are experts at handling such difficult clients and consequently keep the practice bad debts well under control.

Teacher and advisor

Nurses, especially, have these roles, particularly in their nurse's clinics where nutritional, dental and other general advice is given. But all support staff are teaching and advising clients about pet health care, flea control, worming, vaccination and pet travel schemes every day, the list is endless. The vet, of course, gives detailed clinical advice to clients, but the role of support staff in advising clients is large and constantly increasing as veterinary surgeries rely more and more on nurses in particular, to carry out client education and develop new client services.

Artist and designer

Many support staff never realised what artistic talents they had until they were asked to design the front cover of the practice newsletter, or the posters for the client seminar. And their skills may be tested to the full by the monthly displays they are responsible for in the waiting room. Yes, it's support staff again who are responsible for all the floral displays and the green foliage which bedecks the waiting room.

Not everyone has an artistic bent but there are certainly opportunities for those who have or would like to develop them.

Politician and peacekeeper

This is a role support staff take on with both clients and staff.

It is the support staff who usually have to deal with the difficult or angry client, using their skills as politician and peacekeeper.

The client wanting an appointment at 10.30 a.m. on a busy Monday morning, who won't take no for an answer, needs to be persuaded that although he can't have the 10.30 a.m. appointment, he can have one at 12.30 p.m. And that, in any case, this would be much better for Bonzo, as it's his favourite vet who is free then.

The angry client shouting about her unexpectedly large vet's bill needs to be removed from the waiting room and pacified by an experienced member of staff, who uses all the right words and body language to deflate the client's anger.

Political skills come even more to the fore when dealing with other members of staff and veterinary surgeons. It's a fine balancing act, keeping everyone happy, providing clients with appointments and vets with enough free time to make their telephone calls and do their paperwork. The receptionist has to make sure that Mrs. Jones, who always overstays her appointment time, sees her favourite vet, while remembering that he needs to leave early that evening because he has a dental appointment, so it's important they don't book her in as the last appointment at 5.55 p.m. Many is the time when the receptionist will feel she is walking a tightrope, while juggling with at least half a dozen other problems and her skills as a politician are being stretched to the limit.

What support staff say

Support staff from three different surgeries were asked to describe their roles, how long they had worked for the practice and the job they had been doing before.

Pat – Senior Receptionist for 20 years; role involves telephone enquiries, dealing directly with clients in the waiting room, making appointments, selling products, updating client records on the computer and generating computer data; previous job, quality control laboratory assistant in the food industry.

Figure 2   Primary and secondary support staff roles

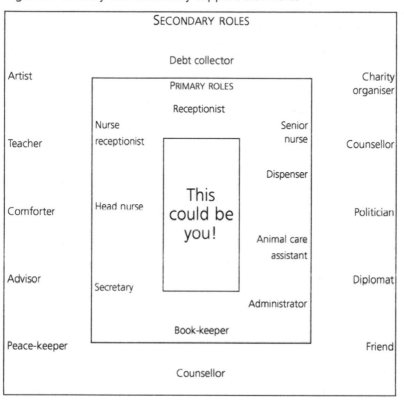

Elaine – **Head Receptionist** for four years; role involves organising
   reception staff and rotas, liaising with practice nurse, sending client
   accounts, liasing with vets and nurses to ensure good communications,
   dealing with account queries; previous job bank clerk/cashier.

Christine – **Staff Supervisor** for seven years; role involves supervising
   smooth running of the surgery, organising staff rotas, reception
   duties, dispensing drugs and helping in the operating theatre;
   previous job, supervisory role with Eastern Electricity.

Alison – **Receptionist** for two years; role involves giving clients advice
   on the phone and in the waiting room, booking appointments, cashing
   up, booking operations and appointments, checking first aid
   equipment, giving first aid talks as the practice first aider, keeping the
   reception area clean and tidy; previous job also veterinary
   receptionist.

Sheila – Office Manager for one year; role involves day to day running of the office, processing all the accounts and calculating VAT; previous job, accounts manager.

Liz – Head Dispenser and Purchasing Officer for seven years; role involves overseeing the running of the dispensary, drug purchasing, stock control, equipment purchase and responsibility for health and safety; previous job, nursing auxillary.

April – Secretary and Administrator for 11 years; role involves practice administration, dealing with personnel problems, doing the practice accounts and organising the health and safety paperwork; previous job, legal secretary for RAF.

Sharon – Practice Secretary for six years; role involves typing, filing, sending client accounts and 'boosters', designing and producing the hospital newsletter and posters, processing drug invoices; previous job, care assistant in nursing home.

Elizabeth – Large Animal Receptionist for seven months; role involves answering telephone, organising the large animal calls and daily farm visits, Ministry of Agriculture paperwork, animal exports, responsibility for fax, photocopying and franking machines, the mail and petty cash; previous job, customer services operator for Nat West Bank.

Denise – Staff Supervisor for 19 years; role involves day to day supervision of staff; previous job, receptionist in the practice.

Margaret – Administrative Assistant for nine years; role involves administering insurance claims, typing, filing, cover for switch board and receptionists, some health and safety risk assessments; previous job dental receptionist.

Summary

- Support staff need to be truly multi-skilled members of the practice team combining the tasks listed in their official job description with the secondary more ephemeral but just as important roles.
- Support staff are all the people in veterinary practice who are not vets, their function is to enable the smooth running of the practice while the veterinary surgeons carry out their clinical role.
- Non-nursing support staff are often older due to the part-time possibilities of the job.
- Support staff need to have good computer skills and a sound basic education.
- A proportion of support staff are recruited from other service industries.
- Support staff must be team members.
- Working in a veterinary surgery means caring for animals and their owners.
- Support staff have to be able to juggle a number of jobs all at the same time.
- Support staff have primary and secondary roles in veterinary practice.

Exercise 1

List the main duties of your job and then list the secondary roles you carry out in your job in the veterinary practice and give examples of what these secondary roles involve.

2

Support staff
and the practice image

The image clients have of their veterinary practice is vital to the success of the practice. They must have a positive image of their practice, seeing it as a friendly welcoming place where they will receive specialist and helpful advice about the care and health of their pet. Pet owners must feel their practice provides a high standard of treatment and care, and be proud to belong as a client of the practice.

Support staff can make or break the practice image by their attitude to, and care of, clients. The practice image is produced by a combination of good client care and quality service, and support staff are important people in the practice providing these two ingredients.

The importance of client care

Client care is important because if we do not care for clients they will go elsewhere and the veterinary practice will not prosper.

Clients provide the only income a practice has and loss of clients means loss of income, and potentially loss of support staff and veterinary jobs.

Satisfied 'well cared for' clients tell others, so good client care is also one of the secrets to good marketing of the practice. It is worth remembering that most clients cannot judge the quality of the veterinary care their animal receives, but they can judge the quality of client care given by the support staff.

Providing the best possible client care is fundamental to the success of the veterinary practice and the job satisfaction of all the staff.

What is a quality service?

A quality service exceeds the expectations of the client. It is giving 101% service rather than 100% service. It is phoning Bonzo's owner to check that he is all right after his castration operation yesterday, or suggesting that he attends the practice older pet clinics now that he is over eight years old, or sending him a birthday card each year.

A quality service might also involve:

- Sending a personal invitation to the practice open day to the top 20% clients.
- Posting client newsletters to bonded clients.
- Remembering to ask Mrs Jones if she had a good holiday.
- Keeping clients informed about the latest flea and worming products.
- Remembering to ask after Mrs Brown's father now he is out of hospital.
- Being able to advise a confused client on the different types of pet insurance.

It is a mixture of quality information provision and more personal client care, which makes the client feel special, and well served by the practice.

Different clients have different perceptions of quality. A service which may be good enough for one client, may not be good enough for another. Support staff should aim to satisfy the highest demands, that way all the clients will be satisfied.

A quality service is one that is always improving and support staff should be playing their part in constantly looking to see where the service to clients can be improved, as these examples show:

- ⇨ If a receptionist notices that more and more clients are requesting late appointments, she should discuss this with her manager or the veterinary surgeon, so that perhaps the practice may introduce later opening hours once or twice a week for these clients.
- ⇨ The receptionist may decide to put the photos clients bring of their pets (which are normally stored in the reception desk drawer) into an album for display in the reception area, or perhaps organise a 'Pets display board' where photos are displayed for fixed periods of time. The pleasure clients will gain from seeing their pets' photos displayed will be enormous and a great benefit to the practice in terms of goodwill and client bonding.

What does the client want?

Top of the list of reasons clients give for choosing a veterinary practice is 'caring staff'. The quality of the clinical care their animal receives is usually taken for granted and it is the other factors like caring staff, clean and pleasant surroundings, efficient service and location which determine the veterinary practice they go to.

The client wants both themselves and their pet to be made to feel special by the practice. This is an important area where support staff can play a major role by providing that special service.

Support staff need to ensure that clients feel that they have had a 'good experience' at the veterinary surgery. Visiting the veterinary surgery should be (as far as is possible if a pet is ill, rather than just having a check up or annual vaccination) a pleasant experience for clients which helps to bond them to the practice. Friendly staff, providing clear and relevant advice in a pleasant atmosphere, together with the expected veterinary expertise, will go a very long way to provide what most clients want from their veterinary practice. And if clients are treated in this way they will naturally assume that their pet will receive the same care and attention if it has to be admitted for an operation or hospitalised. All these factors go towards building the trust and confidence the client is looking for in the veterinary practice and its staff.

What is the role of support staff in client care?

Support staff have the most important role in providing good client care in the veterinary practice. Clients judge the practice even before they walk into the waiting room, by the tidiness of the car park, the signage, the presence of a dog loo and so on. However, once they have entered the waiting room, the first staff they see are the receptionists, and how the receptionist greets the client, is heard answering the telephone, or deals with other clients in the waiting room is vital to the client's perception of the client care the veterinary practice provides.

The receptionist is also often the last member of staff the client sees when leaving the practice. It is this last encounter which they are likely to remember most, so it needs to be a pleasant and comfortable experience, not a fight

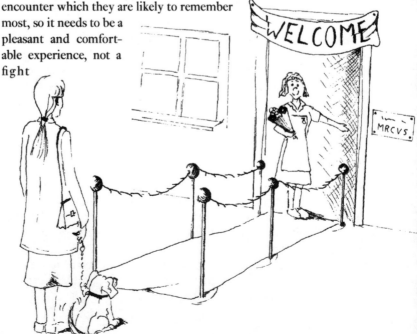

over paying a bill or difficulty in making another appointment.

Clients may be anxious, worried, stressed, annoyed or in other emotional states and it is the receptionist's job to reassure the client, build confidence about the treatment and health of their pet and ensure the client leaves the practice satisfied.

It's a tall order and below are some of the ways to achieve good client care.

Figure 3   What does the client want?

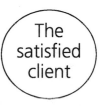

Information about veterinary
  services

Convenient appointment
  times

Made to feel special

Caring, friendly staff and vets

Clean and tidy surgery

Staff they can talk to

The
satisfied
client

Value for money

Good client care

Easy parking

Quality veterinary
products

Reassurance

Helpful staff

The best clinical care
for their pets

First impressions count

Clients judge the practice from the moment they see the building. They judge the state of repair of the premises, the tidiness and cleanliness of the car park and even whether the veterinary surgeon's brass nameplate has been polished in the last month.

However, once they are in the waiting room they have far more areas to judge, and what they see, in their eyes, reflects the standard of service they assume they will receive.

Below are the major areas and aspects of the waiting room which receptionists and support staff should be paying careful attention to.

Smell

Nothing is worse than walking into a veterinary surgery waiting room and being hit by the smell of stale urine. It's not possible to prevent every dog from peeing against the corner of the reception desk or by the pot plant in the entrance, but measures can be taken to eliminate the smell:

⇨ Clean up any mess immediately.

⇨ Have a cloth/mop/disinfectant at hand.

⇨ Clean up the mess with grace, this always impresses the client.

⇨ Use an air freshener, there are many good products on the market, some of which are plugged into an electric socket and can be adjusted to release more or less fragrance.

⇨ Change the matting regularly.

⇨ Have a dog loo in the car park.

Cleanliness

If the waiting room is dirty the client will assume the rest of the practice is the same. Will surgical procedures be of a low standard, will the instruments be clean and what about the kennels? State of the art surgical equipment will be of no value if the client has already lost confidence by looking at the state of the waiting room.

⇨ Clean the floor at least twice a day and also if it gets really dirty in between.

⇨ Keep the windows clean inside and outside, it may not be the receptionist's job to clean the windows but it is her job to inform the manager/partner that they need cleaning.

⇨ The paint work should be clean.

⇨ Chairs should be free from muddy paw prints.

State of repair

It is obviously the responsibility of the management to organise repairs to the practice building but receptionists should be highlighting areas which need attention.

◆ Is the paint work old and peeling?

◆ Are upholstered chairs now torn?

◆ Do the walls need repainting?

◆ Is there still bluetack stuck to the paint work from when the last poster was removed or was the paint also pulled off with the bluetack?

These are all indications to the client that the practice does not really care and certainly doesn't pay attention to detail.

A welcoming waiting room

The client needs to feel welcomed as soon as they enter the waiting room and this is not just by a smiling receptionist, but also by comfortable, pleasant surroundings. It's all in the way the waiting room looks, the colour, the displays, in fact all the areas discussed earlier go to provide either a welcome to the client or a cold negative reception.

A tidy waiting room

Tidiness is another indication of how the practice operates. If the reception desk is strewn with pieces of paper, post-it notes and telephone messages and the notice board behind the desk is so overloaded that it's about to fall off the wall, a client might feel that the rest of the practice functions in the same manner.

⇨ Keep the reception desk tidy at all times; if there really has to be an untidy area due to lack of space make sure the client cannot see it.

⇨ Tidy up magazines and newsletter after clients have read them, preferably store them in magazine racks.

⇨ Store information leaflets in plastic holders – don't have them strewn

over all the available surfaces in the waiting room.
⇨ If there is a children's play area, tidy it up after little Johnny has gone home.

Posters and displays

These can make or break a waiting room. A good display conveys a lot of useful information to clients and can be very successful in promoting new services or products. A badly designed or messy display simply turns the client off and they don't even bother to begin to read it. The support staff and receptionists are usually responsible for designing displays and organising posters in the waiting room and will benefit from following these few golden rules:

⇨ Don't clutter the waiting room with too many posters and displays so that clients 'cannot see the wood for the trees'.
⇨ Don't put posters on the wall without a frame or a glass clip-frame.
⇨ Never, never stick pieces of paper or notices on the walls with bluetack – within days these notices will be sagging and curling at the edges.
⇨ Keep displays simple so that the message is put over to the client.
⇨ Try to theme posters and displays with the time of year, the practice newsletter or a particular practice promotion such as National Pet Week or Pet Smile Week.
⇨ Have the occasional display of 'behind the scenes' photographs – the client rarely sees what goes on past the waiting room, so it can be very worthwhile to display photos of the operating theatre or kennels.

Vegetation

Plants can make the waiting room look very attractive so long as they do not turn it into a jungle. There are really only two rules about plants:
⇨ Better have a few really attractive plants than a dozen indiscriminate

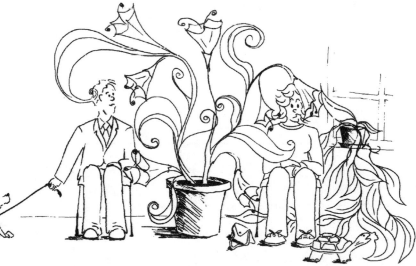

pots of foliage – often one pretty vase of flowers on the reception desk can be sufficient.

⇨ No dead or dying plants – if you can't even keep the plants alive, what can the client expect for the fate of their pet?

The receptionist

The appearance of the receptionist influences clients tremendously. A sloppily dressed receptionist suggests a sloppy service. Many receptionists in veterinary practices wear a uniform and a name badge, which helps clients identify who they are talking to and their role in the practice. Whether or not they wear a uniform, receptionists should look clean and tidy and, like nurses, preferably have long hair controlled so that it does not fall all over the appointment diary when the client is booking their return visit.

Last impressions

Last impressions are just as important as first and the way the client is treated as they prepare to leave the surgery influences their ffnal impression of the surgery and its service.

Figure 4   First and last impressions:
A client's journey through the practice

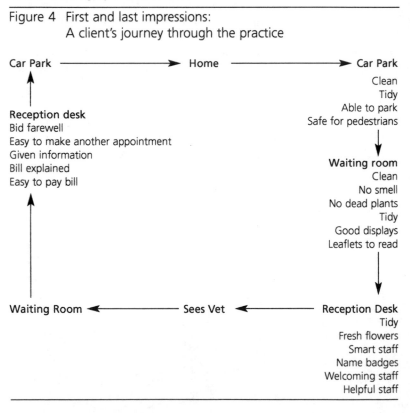

Summary

Some of the factors which influence clients and leave them with good impressions are:

- Not having to queue to pay the bill.
- Being able to pay the bill by credit/debit card.
- The bill is not more than expected (no unpleasant surprises for the client at this stage).
- Ease of making another appointment.
- Receptionist able to provide client with information required in other pet care areas (e. g. pet food, pet insurance).
- Receptionist is cheerful and friendly and says goodbye.
- Client's car is not blocked in buy other cars in the car park.

What support staff say

Q: How does your practice provide good client care?

Christine: I think we pride ourselves on being a friendly practice and treat our clients as important individuals, as well as providing a high standard of veterinary care. We treat our clients as friends.

Denise: By being there at all times and having good and experienced staff.

Alison: By being polite, sympathetic and efficient. We try to consider the client's situation and be understanding and patient, and we are always welcoming and friendly.

Elaine: We have a client newsletter giving seasonal information and details of practice services. We have lunchtime staff meetings on new drugs and services so that we can inform clients properly and we continually appraise our services to ensure we are catering for our clients' needs.

Liz: By ensuring staff are aware of the aims of the practice and by having high standards of treatment, equipment and services.

Exercise 2

List all the different ways you think your practice provides a quality service. Make a second list of extra ways you think a quality of service could be improved.

3

Support staff
and client care skills

The role of the receptionist is fundamental to the overall success of the veterinary practice. As the first and last point of contact for clients, how the receptionist answers the telephone, her attitude and body language, helpfulness and knowledge helps to form the client's lasting impression of the practice.

Support staff working in the reception area require many client care skills.

Greeting the client

The client needs to feel welcomed into the practice. The receptionist may be busy dealing with another client, but as soon as a new client enters the waiting room they should be acknowledged. A quick smile and nod of the head from the receptionist, indicating that they have seen the client and that they will deal with them as soon as possible, may be enough. Or the receptionist may greet the client and ask them to take a seat until she can

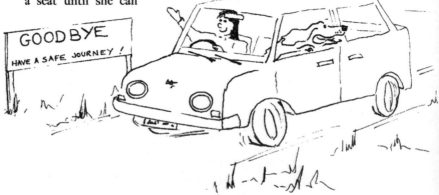

deal with them. The important point to remember is that no one likes to be ignored, especially if they are anxious or stressed.

Greeting a client by name and knowing the name of their pet is essential. If a client has an appointment it is an easy matter for the receptionist to work out who they are when they come into the waiting room, even if they don't immediately recognise them. Many receptionists will admit they find it easier to remember the names of pets than those of owners, especially if they meet the owner and their pet outside the surgery.

Once the client has been welcomed, their appointment should be confirmed and the receptionist should check the client's name, pet's name and the reason for coming to the surgery. If the vet is running late the client should always be informed. Clients don't particularly like to be kept waiting, but not telling them why they are waiting or how long they may have to wait is a recipe for disaster. If it's going to be a long wait offer the client a cup of coffee, an alternative appointment and apologies but don't ignore them, try to make them feel special. However do not be tempted to give away too much information about why the appointments are running late. If there has for example been a road traffic accident brought in which is causing the delay, don't say, 'Sorry for the delay it's because Mrs Blogg's dog has been run over by the coal lorry'.

Don't disclose confidential information to the clients.

Saying farewell to the client is just as important as welcoming them. Their last impression will remain with them, it needs to be a pleasant one. Having taken payment from the client the receptionist should confirm any further

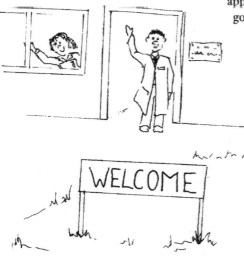

appointment and then say goodbye to the client, again smiling and looking at them – not with their head buried in the appointment book or eyes fixed on the computer screen.

Clients with disabilities may need special consideration. A disablement may be visual and the client has a guide dog, such clients may need help finding a seat and need leading to the consulting room. Other clients may be hard of hearing or have physical or mental disabilities. Receptionists should always make sure they have understood the client's needs and that the client has understood any instructions, information or advice they have been given.

Telephone skills

Poor telephone skills lose clients and potential clients. It is of course important to answer the telephone quickly, but it is even more important how it is answered – the tone of voice, the words used and the information given.

A skilled receptionist will answer the telephone quickly, politely and efficiently, giving and receiving relevant information, and creating business for the practice by making appointments, informing clients of the services and products the practice offers. Below are some of the most important telephone skills support staff require.

▷ Calls should be answered promptly, within three to five rings.

▷ If the receptionist is really busy she should ask the client to hold, but only after having first made sure that the call is not an emergency. If the client is holding they should be returned to every 20–30 seconds.

▷ If the receptionist is already dealing with a client in the waiting room when the telephone rings, they should excuse themselves and ask the client if they could just wait a moment while they answer the telephone.

▷ The caller should be greeted with the accepted practice greeting – 'Good morning this is the ABC Veterinary Practice, how may I help you?' It is helpful if the receptionist also gives her name so that the client knows who they are speaking to.

▷ The receptionist should sound welcoming and positive, speaking clearly and slowly.

▷ The client should be made to feel that the receptionist really wants to talk to them, and not that they are a nuisance.

▷ Smiling as you answer the telephone really does make you sound happier and more welcoming.

▷ The receptionist should listen carefully to the client, make relevant notes and take down information which they may need to pass on. They should read back any message or information the client has given to ensure it has been recorded correctly.

▷ When appointments are booked they should also be read back to the client and the receptionist should be sure that the client has understood any other information which they have been given.

▷ If the receptionist promises to phone the client back they should do so at the promised time. Agreeing a return telephone call from a vet is more difficult, and it is important to give the vet some flexibility if possible unless they set aside a specific time for making telephone calls. The receptionist should make sure they know the practice policy on return telephone calls.

⇨ The client's name and the pet's name should be used when speaking to them – it sounds far more personal.

⇨ If the client is very talkative, (and some certainly are), the receptionist should try to ask questions which steer the client back to the point of the phone call.

⇨ At the end of the call, the client should be thanked by name for calling before the receptionist says goodbye.

A few phrases receptionists should never use when on the telephone are – 'Hang on a minute', 'Just a tick', 'OK', 'Wait a second', 'What was the name again?'

How the receptionist looks, sounds and behaves

Receptionists should dress to portray the correct practice image. They should be smart, tidy and preferably wear a name badge as clients do like to know who they are talking to.

The receptionist should always sound interested in the client's 'problems', and be mindful that the tone of their voice conveys as much information as the words they speak. Smiling at the client will help to relax them and put them at their ease, smiling at someone often makes them smile back! Eye contact should be made with the client to show an interest in them but it is important to remember that prolonged, direct eye contact can be seen as aggressive.

Body language is important, gestures and posture convey all kinds of non-verbal communication. The receptionist should display open body language, no folding of arms, hands on hips or pointing a finger at the client. It is important also not to invade the client's personal space by moving too close and crowding them, this can be both uncomfortable and irritating. It is best to adopt open gestures, a relaxed pose and smile or nod when the client speaks, and maintain good eye contact by looking at their face as a whole rather than staring them fixedly in the eyes. Don't, however, then stare at their nose or right ear instead as they will begin to wonder what is wrong with that particular part of their anatomy!

The receptionist should convey confidence in their role and the way they help and advise the client, this helps to build up trust. For example, if Mrs Smith asks the receptionist how long it will take for her cat Sophie to come round after her spay, the receptionist should be able to reply confidently:

Well, Mrs Smith it normally takes about 30 minutes for cats to come round. But of course every cat is slightly different. Let me give you our

*practice leaflet on cat spays which has more information about the oper-
ation and caring for your pet afterwards.*

Mrs Smith is certainly going to feel that the receptionist knows her job and
understands what will be happening to Sophie. The client does not want
to hear, 'I'm not really sure, it depends, perhaps you should ask the vet'.

Staff in a veterinary practice should be seen as the client's friends –
approachable, helpful, able to give advice and sympathy in appropriate
measures. It is important to show empathy with the client and try to
understand and identify with their feelings. The client needs to feel that
the staff understand their problem, this gives them the confidence and
trust that everything 'will be all right' and their pet will receive the best
treatment. Building up empathy can be difficult especially with awkward
clients, but it is important for staff to try and put themselves in a client's
shoes and look at the situation from their point of view. If, for example,
Mrs Brown has brought her 16 year old cat who has been her only companion for the last five years to be euthanased, the receptionist would not
greet her with a big, happy smile saying, 'Hello, how are you Mrs Brown,
isn't it a lovely day.' She would greet Mrs Brown with a friendly but sympathetic smile and simply say 'Good morning Mrs Brown'.

Sensitive situations

Receptionists are constantly having to deal with sensitive situations and
the example of Mrs Brown and her cat is typical. Other examples might
be:

◆ road traffic accidents (RTAs)
◆ serious illness
◆ lost pets
◆ clients who have genuine difficulties paying their bill, especially
   elderly clients
◆ the sharing out of pets when a marriage breaks up.

Support staff have to be sensitive to all these situations and many others, showing concern, and understanding, but at the same time
maintaining the professionalism and efficiency that the job requires.

The general rule is to show the client that you care while dealing with
them in a professional and businesslike manner.

Booking appointments and operations

One of the primary roles of the receptionist is to provide an efficient booking service for clients, both for appointments and for their pet's operations.
Many practices now use a computer booking system.

Receptionists should be totally familiar with the practice policy on

booking appointments, knowing the policy on:
- length of appointment
- when to give 'long' appointments
- multiple animal booking
- clients arriving with no appointments
- clients wanting to see specific veterinary surgeons
- rest breaks
- catching up time
- extra appointments
- nurse's clinic appointments
- practice nurse appointments
- client appointment cards
- how to deal with appointments when they are running late
- what combination of appointments to book
- what combination of operations to book
- how many operations to book
- emergencies.

They also need to know:
- any client's preference for a particular vet and *vice versa*
- clients who always take up extra time in the consulting room
- any clients who always bring their three children with them
- clients who bring three animals even though they have only booked in one
- which vets are slower or quicker with appointments
- the importance of repeating the time of the appointment to the client, especially over the telephone: 14:30 and 4:30 sound very similar on the phone.

This second list could be endless and varies with every practice but it's all vital information the receptionist needs.

Although nurses may usually talk to clients about pre- and post-operative care for their pets, receptionists have to be familiar with these instructions as they may also be required to advise clients. Receptionists are often asked questions about operations. Although the vet or vet nurse will be able to give a more detailed answer the receptionist should be familiar with the routine operations such as spays, castrations, dentals, so that they can give basic information to the client.

It is very beneficial if support staff have spent time watching operations and having them explained, so that they can talk to the client with some confidence about the procedures. It also makes the whole process far more interesting for the support staff, who can then feel more involved in the whole process of animal admission.

Listening

Listening is an essential skill all veterinary staff must have. To avoid embarrassing and potentially serious mistakes, it is vital to be absolutely sure what the client has said *and* what they want.

Here are just a few of the terms clients used for neutering pets:

◆ seen to
◆ chopped
◆ done
◆ spayed
◆ neutered
◆ sliced
◆ taken away.

The poor receptionist, faced with the plethora of different terms for the same procedure, needs to be absolutely sure they have understood the correct message and should always check with the client exactly what they want. Does 'seen to' for example, mean neutered, vaccinated, or euthanased? Tragedies have happened and it is never worth leave anything to chance. Staff should always double check if they are uncertain.

Providing information

Receptionists are often the client's first port of call for information. There may be a practice nurse who advises clients and nurses running clinics who do the same, but the receptionist needs to be prepared to answer client queries knowledgeably and accurately. The receptionist needs a very wide knowledge of veterinary information to carry out her job effectively. This takes time to learn and the training covered in Chapter 9 will discuss this in more detail. Listed below are just some of the areas on which the receptionist needs to be able to advise clients:

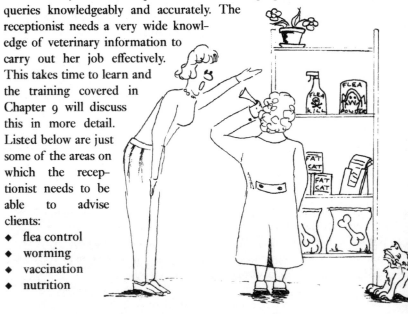

◆ flea control
◆ worming
◆ vaccination
◆ nutrition

- pet insurance
- animal charities
- gestation periods
- tablet administration
- pet products.

Now that pets can be taken abroad on holiday receptionists also need to be able to advise clients on the Pet Passport Scheme and the need for microchipping. They will also have to know about pet export regulations for different countries and the vaccinations and health examinations required pre-export.

Support staff will also need to be able to advise and market to clients practice services such as:-

- nurse's clinics:
  older pet clinics
  puppy clinics and parties
  adolescent pet clinics
  nutrition and weight clinics
- dental clinics
- client seminars
- specialist veterinary services

- dermatology clinics
- alternative medicine
  acupuncture
  holistic and herbal medicine
- information leaflets
- client newsletters
- practice website
- budget payment schemes.

Sales and marketing

Receptionists do have to become involved with selling products and marketing services. I have heard many receptionists say, 'I didn't take this job just to sell pet food or pet insurance.' This may be true but the reality of veterinary practice today is that sales and marketing is an important part of the business of any practice, which must be taken on board by all staff, and should be included in their job description.

Sales

If there is a sales area in the waiting room, part of a receptionist's role is to help clients purchase products they need by providing them with the relevant information about the product. A receptionist should never try to persuade a client to buy something that is not appropriate, the principle is to enable them to purchase products they really need or have decided they want. This may be by explaining to the client the benefits of a balanced dried food diet or the fun lots of clients' pets have had from a particular toy.

Marketing

Marketing the services of the practice is essential today when practices face increasing competition. The purpose of marketing is to make sure the client stays with the practice, to attract new clients and to create more business from the clients that the practice already has. The receptionist is marketing the practice every day. At the basic level it is by looking smart, being helpful and giving clients a good impression of the practice. At a more complex level marketing is implementing programmes, ideas and procedures to encourage a profitable relationship between the practice and the clients, and includes the services the practice offers, the fees charged and the promotion and advertising of the practice.

Everyone in the practice is involved in marketing at some level but receptionists are in an ideal position to help promote the practice services, by talking to clients in the waiting room and on the telephone. So if a client telephones or calls in to enquire about the price of a cat spay, the receptionist should not just simply quote the price, but should explain the procedure, and the care the practice provides, how the vets like to see the cat first, how the nurse will telephone the day after the operation to check that everything is all right. They are showing the client why they should come to this practice rather than the 'one down the road'. Sales and marketing are dealt with in detail in Chapter 5.

Debt control

This is definitely one of the less popular support staff roles. In an ideal world every client would pay their bill before they left the surgery, sadly we do not live in such a world and the receptionist has to deal with many and varied excuses from clients for not paying their bills. Just a few common examples are:

Forgotten my purse.
Giro comes tomorrow.
I will come back with money on Thursday when I've been paid.
My husband will pay.
My wife will pay.
Mum has sent me to collect Bonzo.
I'm just collecting the cat for my sister, she will pay.
I'll pay when the stitches are taken out.
I'll pay at the end of the treatment.
I'll bring the money tomorrow.
The bill is much higher than the estimate, I'm not paying all this.

And then of course there are the sensitive situations such as:

- RTAs
- euthanasias
- genuine cases of hardship.

For the client who is deliberately trying to avoid payment there are a number of replies and techniques the receptionist can use to encourage the handing over of payment.

⇨ 'Well Mrs Brown, what time shall I tell the receptionist on duty

tomorrow that you will call with the payment?'
➪ 'I'm sorry but we require payment today, not when the stitches are taken out.'
➪ 'If you have forgotten your purse, do you have a credit or debit card with you or perhaps your cheque book? We can accept all these kinds of payment.'
➪ 'Here is the bill for Ben's operation, please give it to your Mum and tell her we will telephone her tomorrow about when she is going to pay.'

Receptionists need to be positive, firm and assertive about asking clients to pay, but they do have to use their discretion and no one should be demanding payment from a distraught client whose treasured pet has just been euthanased.

However there needs to be a set practice policy on following up clients who have not paid at the time. With euthanasias the policy is often to send the bill a week after the euthanasia, and for any non-payers there is usually a set procedure of letters, telephone calls and debt collecting agency referral.

Below are a few client care skills which will help to ensure payment at the time of treatment.
➪ Ask the clients how they would like to pay before they have had the consultation or operation.
➪ Always have a notice in the waiting room stating that payment must be at the time of treatment. You can refer to it if there is a problem and the client has at least been informed what the practice conditions are.
➪ Overestimate rather than underestimate a potential bill – never give the client unpleasant surprises.
➪ Make sure you have included the VAT on the bill before you tell the client how much they owe, but do tell them the VAT element of the bill, after all the practice does not keep this money.
➪ Give advice on the help animal charities give to clients who have difficulty paying.
➪ Encourage clients to take out pet insurance.
➪ Always thank the client for paying the bill.
➪ Offer instalment payments only if it is the practice policy.

Debt control is covered in greater detail in the finance section of Chapter 5.

Being a team member

Veterinary practices only work well if all the staff and vets work as a team. The practice should be seen as one large team within which there are a number of smaller teams comprising, vets, nurses, receptionists and admin staff. Each individual team must work well together, communicating, co-operating and helping each other and they must also communicate with the other teams so that the practice operates efficiently and effectively. Teamwork results in greater achievements and success through people working together rather than as individuals and provides greater job satisfaction for all concerned.

Outside the practice

It is inevitable that support staff will meet clients outside the practice. The scenario often goes like this.

Mrs Bloggs meets Mary the Receptionist in the supermarket on a Saturday morning.

Mrs Bloggs: 'Hello Mary how are you?'

Mary: 'Fine thank you, how is Bonzo?

Mrs Bloggs: 'Wonderful, but you know I do think that I was charged too much for Bonzo's operation last month, and Fifi doesn't seem to be any better yet she's still limping, what do you think might be wrong?'

Mary: 'Well...'

Mrs Bloggs: 'My other cat Rosie is scratching her ears all the time, do you think I should treat her for fleas, which product should I get?'

Mary: ...!

Sounds familiar?

Support staff are representing the practice even when they are off duty, but this does not mean they have to give help or advice to clients like Mrs Bloggs. Mary's answer to Mrs Bloggs and others like her should be:

Well if you're worried Mrs Bloggs, phone the surgery on Monday morning and I'm sure that we will be able to help you.

Support staff should not get involved in practice matters when they are off duty, it can be a recipe for disaster. We all need our free time away from work even if clients sometimes think otherwise.

What prevents good client care

A breakdown in any one of the many areas of client service we have discussed will reduce the standard of client care. But the main reason for failure to produce good client care is lack of communication, either between staff and the client or between the staff themselves.

Listening skills play an important part here. Staff should listen to the client and be sure they understand what is being said or asked and what the client really wants. Staff must always make sure that the client understands the information they have been given.

Passing information on to other staff accurately and efficiently is vital,

Figure 5 The components of successful client care

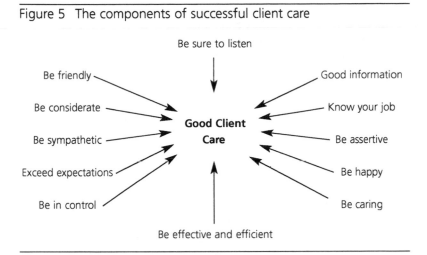

post-it notes should not be lying around the reception desk for two days before they reach the person the message was for! Communication with other members of the team is essential, especially as support staff are often part-time and do not see each other every day. A good system for staff who do not see each other regularly is to have a notebook in which to record all messages and information that needs to be seen by other staff members, this book should always be kept in the same place for all staff to refer to. It is very useful to have changeover periods when, for example in the reception team, the receptionist going off duty has time to talk to the receptionist coming on duty about what happened on her shift and what items need to be dealt with. The message is communicate, communicate, communicate.

Other important reasons for poor client care can be:-

⇨ Poorly trained staff – who are unable to answer client queries efficiently.

⇨ Lack of attention to detail – sometimes because there is no formal detailed practice policy or staff training on how to carry out a procedure. It is so often the little things that count, doing everything else well but then forgetting to say goodbye to the client or not phoning back as they expected at a specific time; they will be what the client remembers of the practice.

⇨ Poor teamwork – this goes along with poor communication, but the members of the team must work together as a group and not against each other as individuals.

Think of the team involved in an operation:

the receptionist who books the operation

the nurse who admits the animal
the vet who carries out the operation
the nurse who provides post op. nursing care
the receptionist who answers the client's query about how the operation has gone
the nurse who discharges the animal.

All these people must work together. The receptionist must book accurately and check that there is enough space in the operating timetable. The nurse who admits must take and communicate the correct details about the animal to the vet, who in turn must inform the nurse of any special care for the animal and what to say to the client. The receptionist answering the client's telephone call must have been given an up-to-date report of the animal's condition and the discharging nurse must be familiar with how the operation went and be able to pass on relevant information to the client. Any one of these people can disrupt the teamwork by not playing their part in the team process.

▷ Not enough staff. – Clients receive a very bad impression of the practice if they see too few staff rushing around trying to do too many jobs. They will be left with a feeling of nervousness and insecurity about how their pet will be treated.

▷ Clinical treatment considered more important than client care. – The clinical treatment of a client's pet is of course absolutely essential, but without the client care skills to accompany it, a client will lose confidence in the practice and seek a more caring replacement.

At the end of the day veterinary practice staff have to show the client how much they care for the pet, and how much they care about providing the client with an excellent service. The well-known phrase, 'they don't care how much you know, until they know how much you care' rings very true.

Summary

- Support staff need a large variety of client-care skills: the correct greeting of clients, good telephone skills, efficient booking of appointments, appropriate body language, ability to listen, handle sensitive situations and market the practice to the client.
- Client care skills still need to be used outside the practice.
- Support staff must be good team members.
- Poor communication is the greatest factor in preventing good client care.
- Poor teamwork, insufficient staff and an over-reliance on clinical skills without client care skills also contribute to a poor client service.

What support staff say

Q: How do you personally provide good client care?

Christine: 'I try to ensure that any grievances which arise are dealt with straight away and that enough time is given to every client so that they have time to discuss their problems. I recently had an owner who had a week's course of tablets to give to her very unco-operative cat, she was finding it almost impossible to give the tablets and was becoming very frustrated and upset. I arranged with her to come in daily to see me to give the cat his tablets. She was very happy with this arrangement and I got satisfaction from helping her.'

Elaine: ' I always try to be professional, polite, cheerful and smiling. I try to pay attention to detail and always follow up client queries and complaints. I try to make sure the client feels important and valued. I believe that clients not only bond with the vet, they also bond with the people they regularly deal with – us, the receptionists. Let's face it, no one wants to sit in a crowded waiting room looking at a sour-faced receptionist.

There have been occasions when I have had to speak to bereaved owners regarding cremation arrangements. I have always made a point of allowing myself plenty of time to talk and listen to them – you simply cannot rush a person at this sad time. I always let the clients know they can talk to me if they need to and I can always put them in touch with a bereavement counsellor if their need is great.

In fact, last August, I had to speak to one such client. Her pet had died just before a bank holiday and she wanted to take her pet to the local pet crematorium. She needed some reassurance about the procedure and because I had actually been to see the crematorium on a trip arranged by the practice, I was able to put her mind at rest.

She telephoned me last October to say that she was sorry she had not been in touch earlier but it had taken her quite a while to get over her pet's death. The purpose of her call was to thank me for spending the time listening. I felt that I had done something really worthwhile.'

Exercise   3

1   Think of some of the excuses your clients have made for not paying their bill and devise replies which would encourage them to pay at the time of treatment.

2   What would you say to Mrs Bloggs on page 32 to reassure her?

4

Assertiveness and dealing with difficult clients

Dealing with clients on a daily basis as well as working in a busy and sometimes stressful environment can be hard work. Difficult clients and colleagues can begin to wear some members of staff down to the point where they stop enjoying their job.

The ability to be assertive or at least use some assertiveness techniques to help overcome some of the daily stress-making situations can be tremendously helpful.

Assertiveness techniques

Being assertive enables support staff to handle any encounter with confidence and efficiency. Confrontation can be handled better and life becomes less stressful. Assertiveness gives greater self esteem and confidence and makes it easier to prevent oneself from being manipulated by both clients and staff. It allows a person to be in control.

Some people are naturally assertive, but those who are not certainly benefit from attending assertiveness courses.

When people learn how to be assertive they experience benefits such as:
- feeling less stressed
- being more tactful
- handling confrontations more easily
- greater self-confidence
- feeling better about themselves and other people
- being able to resist other people's attempts at manipulation
- better communication skills
- feeling in control.

So how can someone who is not assertive find more confidence in dealing with people? The first thing to understand is that we do not all have the same personality or the same ability to be assertive. Most people fall into three main behaviour/personality types:

1 aggressive
2 assertive
3 passive.

This can be illustrated by the answers to the following question:

Please can you help me to carry some sacks of dog food from the store room to the waiting room?

Aggressive answer: 'No, do it yourself I'm far too busy.'

Assertive answer: 'I'm really busy just now, but I can help you in 20 minutes.'

Passive answer: 'Oh, I was just about to do this lab test, but OK, I'll come and help you.'

The aggressive answer is usually said with excessive eye contact, perhaps leaning towards the other person and with a stern or angry expression. Aggressive behaviour is characterised by being:

♦ frightening
♦ loud
♦ threatening
♦ belligerent
♦ unpredictable.

And the receiver of this behaviour, the client or other member of staff, reacts by being:

♦ hurt
♦ resentful
♦ afraid
♦ defensive
♦ aggressive.

The assertive answer is usually said in a rational calm manner in a neutral tone of voice and with good, but not excessive, eye contact. Assertive behaviour is characterised by being:

♦ honest
♦ positive
♦ direct
♦ firm
♦ respectful of others.

And the receiver of this behaviour reacts by being:

♦ respectful

- understanding
- compliant.

The passive answer is usually said without much eye contact in a quiet hesitant voice. Passive behaviour is characterised by being:

- apologetic
- opting out
- weak
- avoiding confrontation.

And the receiver of this behaviour reacts by being:

- exasperated
- resentful
- frustrated
- manipulative.

Behaving assertively starts with thinking assertively so let's look briefly at ways in which the foundations of assertiveness can be laid.

Think assertively by thinking in a positive way about how to deal with a situation and what you want from it. Consider both your rights and those of the other person. We all have the right to be treated with respect, to be listened to, to sometimes put ourselves first and to occasionally make mistakes. Asserting some of these rights and accepting they also exist for others will help assertive behaviour.

There are many assertiveness techniques which can be used but these are the most important.

Stay in control of your feelings

Staying in control of your feelings is essential if you are to achieve a positive result from an encounter with a client or another member of staff. Do not get angry or emotional, however upset the other person may be. Stay calm and reasonable and you will gain control of the situation and achieve what you want from it.

Stand your ground

Don't allow others to persuade you to change your mind or do something you don't want to just so that you can avoid a difficult situation. If you say no, you must mean it, unless there are very special circumstances for you changing your mind.

Maintain good eye contact

Maintaining good eye contact is important. Someone whose eyes are always downcast or who seems to be unable to look at the person they are dealing with often appears submissive and compliant. Good eye contact suggests a positive and confident person who is not afraid and who will not be intimidated. Don't however stare intently at someone for any length of time, as this can be disconcerting and interpreted as aggressive.

Adopt a neutral tone of voice

A neutral tone of voice when others are raising theirs and becoming emotional allows you to be seen to be in control. By maintaining a neutral tone you are not aggravating or intimidating the other person and you are avoiding escalating the situation further.

Adopt an open posture

An open posture indicates friendliness and a willingness to listen. Body language has a great effect on the people you are communicating with (the phrase 'actions speak louder than words' is very true). If you fold your arms and lean forwards you will appear aggressive and threatening and probably cause the other person to do the same, increasing the tension between you. Standing with your arms by your sides, hands slightly raised shows openness and a willingness to listen and help.

Be able to say no

Assertiveness means being able to say no and mean it. It is not easy saying no to difficult clients or persistent colleagues, but say no you must. Adopt the 'broken record' technique of repeating the same message using a variety of words and answers:

> *'No, I can't.'*
> *'No, I am unable to do that.'*
> *'It's not possible.'*
> *'I can't help just now.'*
> *'I'm sorry but that is against our practice policy.'*
> *'I don't think that is possible but I will discuss it with my colleagues.'*
> *'I'll have to discuss that request with the practice manager.'*

Figure 6   Techniques of assertiveness

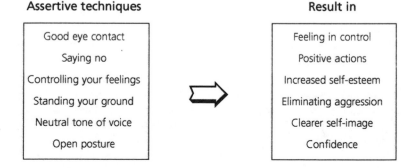

Let's look at an example of how to use these techniques.

Mr Green comes into the surgery on a busy Monday morning with his bulldog, Beano and wants an appointment at 11.00 a.m. There are no appointments until 12.30 p.m. and Beano is not ill, he only needs his annual booster.

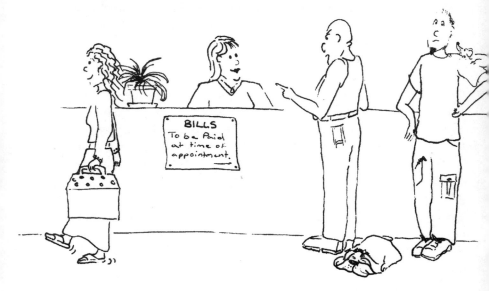

Mr. Green starts to get angry because he cannot have the 11.00 a.m. appointment he wants, but you **stay in control of your feelings**. Remaining calm and polite, you don't get upset or aggressive even though Mr Green, who is by now certainly not in control of his feelings, is really getting to you. **You stand your ground** by refusing to make an exception for Beano by 'squeezing him in' at 10.55 a.m. but offer two alternative appointments at 12.40 p.m. and 12.50 p.m. All the time you are talking to Mr Green you **maintain good eye contact** which helps to reinforce the fact that what you are saying you mean. Despite the fact that Mr Green has raised his voice by three decibels and is quite angry, you maintain a **calm neutral tone of voice** even though you would love to shout back. You are still in control and what's more Mr Green can now see this.

Although Mr Green is becoming agitated, starting to clench his fists and leaning over the counter, you still **maintain an open posture** towards him so that he can see that he is not intimidating you. You have been **able to say no**, calmly and politely and with authority:

We can't see Beano at 11.00 a.m. but we can see him at 12.40. There are no appointments until then. And I'm afraid we can't squeeze him in at 10.55.

Dealing with difficult clients

Working in any service-based business involves dealing with difficult clients on a fairly regular basis. There is no doubt that clients in a veterinary practice can be just as difficult as those in any other small business. But just what is a 'difficult' client? Do the perceptions and attitude of the support staff colour their judgement of some of the so-called difficult people?

There are of course difficult and awkward clients, but there are others who staff see as difficult and therefore treat as such before any real difficulties arise. Let's look first however at the categories of client who we all accept as difficult.

There are many varieties of difficult client but there are three main types:

◆ the complainer
◆ the non-payer
◆ the aggressive client.

The complainer

Most complaints arise from poor communication between the client and the veterinary practice. For example, Mr Alan Black and Mr Arnold Black both have golden labradors called Ben. Mr Alan Black lives at 12 Elm Drive while Mr Arnold Black lives at 21 Elm Drive. Sadly Mr Alan Black's labrador had to be euthanased and we all know that, although unforgivable, how easy it will be in these circumstances to confuse the two Bens. So that when booster-reminder time comes around, it's the wrong Ben whose booster reminder drops through the letter box. Mr Alan Black now has a justified complaint, as has Mr Arnold Black who has not received a reminder at all.

If a client has a justified complaint the following steps should be taken:

↪ Listen without interruption.
↪ Don't get defensive.
↪ Express sympathy.
↪ Ask questions to enable you to understand the problem.
↪ Find out what the client wants.
↪ Explain what you can do.
↪ Discuss alternatives and agree action.
↪ Take the action IMMEDIATELY.
↪ Apologise.
↪ Exceed expectations.

It's worth noting that 70% of clients with grievances will stay with the practice if efforts are made to remedy the complaint and that 95% will stay if the complaint is rectified on the spot.

Some clients will unfortunately complain whatever you do, they are professionals in the complaint stakes. For them nothing will ever be right and if they really cause problems the partners or practice manager may have to consider removing them from the client list.

The non-payer

These clients are the bane of veterinary receptionists' lives. They always have a reason for not paying their bill at the time. Some of the many and varied reasons for not paying were given in Chapter 3 (page 30).

At the end of the day there are really only four main ways of dealing with these clients although hundreds have been tried by all veterinary practices:

⇨ Withhold non-essential drugs – with the permission of the vet.

⇨ Withhold non-essential treatment – again, at the discretion of the vet, as this is likely to be contentious.

⇨ Send their account to a debt-collecting agency or work with a solicitor to recover the debt. – This procedure is not especially successful but does show the client and other potential non-payers that you do pursue the debts.

⇨ Consider removal from the client list.

The aggressive client

Thankfully this type of client is not common in veterinary practices, but they do exist and most support staff can give at least one example of an aggressive client they have had to deal with.

Some people are naturally more aggressive than others, but the kind of client aggression which may be seen is normally due to:

◆ anger
◆ upset
◆ surprise
◆ stress
◆ drink
◆ drugs
◆ just a really 'bad hair day'.

Many veterinary practices have panic buttons or alarms at the reception desk which can be used to call assistance. A telephone should always be close at hand for receptionists to call the police in cases of real danger and the practice should have a written policy or procedure to follow with aggressive or violent clients.

Here are a number of do's and don'ts when it comes to dealing with aggressive clients that all support staff should follow.

Do:

⇨ Appear calm.

⇨ Listen.

⇨ Avoid prolonged eye contact.
⇨ Take care with tone of voice.
⇨ Negotiate.
⇨ Aim for a win/win situation.
⇨ Keep your distance.

Don't

⇨ Overreact.
⇨ Argue or threaten.
⇨ Get angry yourself.
⇨ Raise your voice.
⇨ Make empty threats – if you threaten to call the police do so.
⇨ Block the exit.
⇨ Make physical contact.

Staff attitudes to difficult clients

Staff attitudes can often colour the judgement of clients and sometimes create a 'difficult' client from a perfectly normal pleasant member of the public.

Staff perceptions – What do we see

The following comments are likely to have been made by most veterinary staff at some time:

Oh no, it's Mrs Jones with her budgie, she's always difficult.
It's that chap with the spiky hair and ring in his eyebrow, he's bound to be awkward.
Mrs Hill is here; she was really difficult last Monday, so watch out.

It's easy to make assumptions about clients and because they have been difficult before expect them to be difficult again. Sometimes it's hard for staff not to be prejudiced against clients because of the way they dress or look. Every client should be viewed afresh each time they come into the waiting room – however difficult this may be.

The hidden agenda

Staff only see the very top of a client's agenda – most of the client's feelings, emotions and worries are beneath the surface. Figure 7, over the page, shows the hidden agenda most clients have.

When a client is in the veterinary practice support staff see them behave and respond in a certain way. However there are all sorts of unseen motives, attitudes, feelings and problems – the hidden agenda – which make them behave in the way they do.

For example:

Mrs Smith has an appointment for 10 a.m. but the appointments are running 10 minutes late. Then at 10.10, just as she is about to see the vet, a

RTA is rushed in. Mrs Smith is told that unfortunately her appointment will be delayed for a further 15 minutes. She is offered apologies, a cup of coffee and an alternative appointment but she refuses all these and storms out of the waiting room. What the receptionist has seen is Mrs Smith's behavioural response to a situation and the receptionist probably thinks it is an unreasonable response. However the receptionist does not know Mrs Smith's hidden agenda, which could be any of the following.

Problem – Her husband is going into hospital this afternoon and she is worried; the final demand for the electricity bill arrived this morning and the car broke down on the way to the surgery.

Feelings – Mrs Smith has been very depressed since the death of her mother and is on anti-depressants. It took her a great deal of strength to make herself take her pet to the surgery this morning and face so many people, and having to wait was just more than she could cope with.

Attitude – Mrs Smith doesn't like ginger haired people because they remind her of her sister whom she hasn't spoken to for 10 years. The receptionist had bright ginger hair.

Motive – Mrs Smith is simply attention-seeking.

Figure 7 The hidden agenda

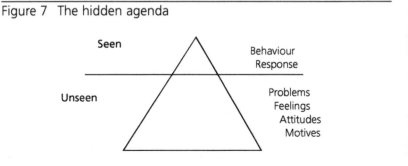

The receptionist is probably never going to know what Mrs Smith's hidden agenda was. But it's highly likely she had one. The point is that support staff dealing with clients need to be aware that clients may have all sorts of reasons for behaving as they do. By appreciating this, it may help support staff to stay calmer and possibly deal better with some of the difficult situations. After all how many of us have not been a 'Mrs Smith'?

Creating the difficult client

Sometimes staff unwittingly make clients difficult by triggering a reaction. It may be by:

⇨ Making an excuse instead of apologising – *We were really busy yesterday*.

⇨ Being defensive – *It wasn't my fault.*

⇨ Adopting an aggressive/unpleasant attitude – *Don't blame me.*

⇨ Blaming someone else for a mistake – *I wasn't here yesterday; it must have been Mary who made the mistake.*

⇨ Forgetting the client's name, or worse, the pet's name.

⇨ Calling the pet by the wrong name.

The transaction between the client and the staff

The behaviour and body language of support staff, in their transaction with the client, will consciously or unconsciously affect the client. If the receptionist smiles at the client, the client will probably smile back; if they frown at the client then the client is likely to frown back. The diagram below shows how positive and negative transactions affect the way people react to each other.

Figure 8 Transactions with clients

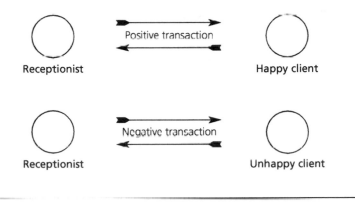

Summary

- Support staff attitudes to, and perceptions of, clients can play an important role in the relationship a client has with the surgery. It is also worth remembering that, although we all complain about difficult clients, 85% of veterinary practice clients are perfectly happy with the practice and its services and never complain.

- There are three main types of behaviour: assertive, aggressive and passive. Being assertive helps you to handle encounters and situations with confidence.

- The main assertive techniques are staying in control of your feelings, standing your ground, maintaining good eye contact, adopting a neutral tone of voice, keeping an open posture and being able to say no.

- Assertiveness results in feeling in control, being positive, increased self-esteem, avoiding aggressive behaviour, a clearer self-image and greater self-confidence.
- There are three main types of difficult client: the complainer, the non-payer and the aggressive client.
- Staff attitudes and perceptions can create 'difficult' clients.
- Clients have hidden agendas which make them behave in the way they do.
- Staff behaviour can sometimes make clients difficult.

What support staff say

Q: What is a 'difficult' client?

Christine: 'An abusive client, a non-payer and one who is difficult to please.'

Pat: 'One who argues over the bill, is rude or abusive, or habitually turns up late and insists on being seen immediately.'

Elaine: 'No client should actually be a difficult client. They are usually people who have misunderstood something or have been misinformed.'

Q: How do you deal with difficult clients?

Christine – 'Let them let off steam, listen but don't argue, ensure that their grievance is dealt with straight away, remain pleasant at all times.

I recently had a client who ran up a bill of over £100 and then rang up to arrange for vaccinations for her two puppies. I explained that until at least £100 had been paid off her bill we could not undertake any further work. She duly arrived and reluctantly handed over the required amount and promised to pay the remainder, which she did after the second vaccination. A subtle mention of the debt collecting agency had the desired effect in this case, the client paid her bill and still stayed on good terms with the practice.'

Elaine: 'Let them vent their anger. Once they have had their say and calmed down I try to clarify their query or complaint. And then resolve the problem; either immediately or explaining exactly what I am going to do and when, ensuring a realistic time scale so that I can meet my promise.

I can think of one of our bonded clients who always likes to see the same vet. She is quite demanding, leaving messages for the vet to telephone her and wanting appointments at short notice – she always thinks her cats are suffering from life threatening illnesses.

A little while ago she called the surgery to make an appointment and was told there was not one available until 11.40 unless she could come in the next 10 minutes. A few minutes later I received a very irate phone call from this lady complaining of the way she had been spoken to. Mindful of the fact that she is a good client, plus the fact that she was likely to tell all and sundry how rude we were, I decided to try some damage limitation. I arranged for her to see a different vet in half an hour, while reinforcing the fact that the receptionist who answered the phone had been correct in saying that the lady's favourite vet was unable to see her.

This lady has health problems, her life revolves around her cats and their (apparent) health problems. She goes through phases of being in and out of the surgery several times a week for many weeks at a time and, as you might expect, her cats are extremely stressed and suffer from bowel and skin problems. It is for this reason that many of the staff find her difficult. I try to take time to talk to her and, because she feels she can talk to me, I am able to persuade her to wait for appointments. She believes I help her as much as I can — that's all it takes, a little understanding.'

Liz: 'I listen to what they are trying to say and use the words "I know how you must be feeling". I remain polite and smile and always try not to be provoked. When I know what the problem is I do my best to sort things out or go and speak to a supervisor.'

Margaret: 'There is one of our clients who is quite disturbed and very difficult to deal with. One day she sat in our surgery for an hour with her cat and spent her time telling the other clients how awful we were. Some of us find her quite frightening. Recently I began to think that this situation was really silly and I made an effort to talk to her and find out some of her problems. Now I am one of the people she asks for when she calls, and she has a much better relationship with us all in reception. What it needed was a little personal care and understanding.'

Pat: 'I can give an example of a client who was complaining about the cost of having an animal treated who became quite personal and abusive. I calmly waited for him to finish speaking which they always do when they run out of steam and then positively dealt with the situation, explaining each and every item which he had been charged for. Once he understood the costs he calmed down and paid. This client still comes to the practice and we regard him now as one of our bonded clients.'

Exercise 4

Mrs. Green is insistent that she stay with her dog Bessie while it is prepared for a bitch spay and while the operation is being carried out. She says she won't leave Bessie for the op. if she can't be with her. Think of as many ways as you can of saying no to Mrs. Green

5

Support staff and money

Money plays an important part in many support staff roles. It may be as
a receptionist taking money from clients and cashing up at the end of
each day;
a member of the admin. staff banking or reconciling bank accounts with
petty cash;
the member of staff responsible for purchase orders and stock control;
as a practice manager or administrator who has to manage the money of
the practice.
Money matters and support staff can be split into four main categories

- taking in the money
- paying out money
- spending money
- managing the money.

Taking the money

This is the major role for support staff. A receptionist must be able to provide, either manually or by computer, client invoices for payment at the
time of treatment and accounts for monthly payment. Receipts, computer
generated or handwritten, also need to be provided. (see figures 9 and 10)
There must be efficient, accurate handling and recording of payments in
whatever form they are made – cash, cheque, credit or debit card. At the
end of every day cashing-up and reconciling the till must be carried out
accurately.

Invoices and receipts
An invoice is a statement of work carried out or products supplied, or
both, and the money owed for this service. All clients must be supplied
with an invoice. This may be automatically generated by the computer at

the end of the consultation and printed in reception for the receptionist to give to the client before they leave. If the practice is not computerised, the receptionist will hand-write the invoice, listing details of consulting fees and drugs from the client's record. The completed invoice must show the client's name, pet's name and address, the practice name and address and the practice VAT registration number and details of the money owed. The computer will automatically put value-added tax (VAT) onto all those items which are not VAT exempt, but if the invoice is manually generated the receptionist will have to calculate VAT. VAT must be charged on all services, medicines and pet foods and products. Currently the VAT rate for these items is at 17½%.

VAT is calculated as follows:

Cost of item/service $\qquad = £12.00$

VAT at 17½% $\qquad \dfrac{£12.00 \times 17.5}{100} \quad = £\ 1.96$

Total cost $\qquad = £13.96$

Normally the VAT charged on each item should be shown separately on the invoice. A receipt should always be given to clients when they pay their bills. This may be simply a 'Received with Thanks' stamped onto the bill which is dated and signed, or it may be a separate receipt manually or computer generated.

Clients pay their bills in a variety of ways:

♦ cash
♦ cheque
♦ debit card
♦ credit card.

Increasingly debit and credit cards are being used in preference to cash and cheques.

Cash is the simplest

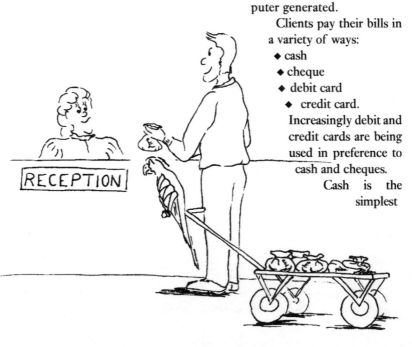

Figure 9 Handwritten Invoice

THE VETERINARY SURGERY

Inv. No. **475**

ANY STREET, ANY TOWN
Tel 01345 67892 Fax. 01345 678 93 email: anyvet@aol.com

INVOICE   Vat Reg. No. 173 46589 26

Invoice to:

Mrs A Brown, 23 Green Street, Anytown

TAX POINT	DESCRIPTION	£ p	VAT at 17.5%
24-3-01	2 bags dog food	16.40	3.27

SUB-TOTALS   16.40   3.27

AMOUNT PAYABLE   £   19.67

---

method of payment, but as veterinary costs rise clients do not always carry
sufficient cash to pay for operations and expensive treatments. Handling
cash requires accuracy and care, so that correct change is given to clients
and the till balances at the end of the day.

Cheques (see figure 11) should only be accepted when a client can provide
a valid cheque guarantee card, although for large amounts the card may not
guarantee the full sum written on the cheque. It is important to write the
card details on the back of the client's cheque. Also to make sure the cheque
is correctly filled in with the right payee, date, the amount written in words
and figures, make sure these amounts are the same – a common mistake
made when writing cheques – and, of course, signed. For the staff who are
responsible for banking, incorrectly filled in cheques are one of their greatest bug bears. Returning cheques to clients because the date was wrong or

Figure 10   Computer-generated invoice

Any Veterinary Group

The Veterinary Surgery   VAT. Reg.No. 173 46589 26
Any Street, Any Town
Tel. 01345 67892 Fax. 01345 67892 e.mail:anyvet@aol.com

Mrs A Brown
23, Green Street   **With reference to:** Paddy 9275
Anytown

Date 31.03.01   **Invoice No.** 37465

Date	Description	Fees	Drugs	Vat	Total
03.03.01	1st FELV Vacc		21.83	3.82	25.65
26.03.01	Cat castrate	17.50		3.06	46.21

WORK DONE THIS MONTH		39.33
VAT (at 17.5%)		6.88

TOTAL FOR THIS MONTH   46 21
TOTAL PAYMENTS THIS MONTH   00.00
TOTAL AMOUNT NOW DUE   46.21

- -

PLEASE CUT OFF THIS REMITTANCE SLIP AND RETURN IT WITH YOUR PAYMENT

Name	Mrs A Brown	**a/c ref**	:	9275
	23, Green Street	**Date**	:	31.03.01
	Anytown	**Due**	:	46.21

they forgot to sign the cheque is a time-consuming business.

Debit cards come in a variety of forms, Switch being one of the common-est. When a debit card is used the client's money is transferred directly from their bank account into the practice bank account. This process normally takes two or three days. The debit card will not work if the client does not have enough money in their bank account.

The main credit cards are; Access, Visa, Mastercard and American

Express. When a credit card is used the amount of money paid is added to the client's credit card account. At the end of the month the client will receive a credit card statement listing all the card transactions and showing the total amount the client now owes on the account. The veterinary practice receives payment from the client credit card account within two or three days of the card being used at the practice.

Most banks now provide electronic credit/debit card machines to businesses through which the clients' cards are passed with details processed electronically. Printout slips are produced which the client must sign and both they and the practice keep a copy.

However the client pays, the transaction must be recorded in the till so that cashing up can be carried out accurately.

Under some circumstances the practice may agree to clients paying bills by direct debit or standing order, or paying off debts by instalments. These systems can cause more work for receptionists but do at least ensure money is paid by the client. Standing orders are agreed fixed amounts paid from the client's bank account at regular intervals into the practice account. Direct debits are also paid from the client's account into the practice account. The amount paid in this case will vary according to the amount the client owes each month and the practice will adjust the money requested from the client's account accordingly. In both cases careful administration of these processes is required, so that client's veterinary

Figure 11   A cheque

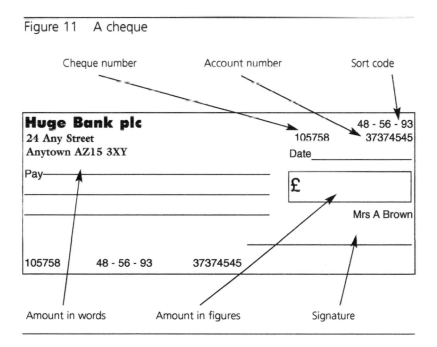

accounts are credited with the payments. Good communication is also needed between receptionist and the person administering the practice bank accounts.

Some practices allow clients, who find it difficult to pay large amounts for treatments all at once, to pay their bills by instalments. This requires the receptionist to keep careful records of how much is owed, what the instalments are and how often they are paid. The payments must be recorded on the client record, and payment defaults need to be noted and dealt with. Instalment payment is time consuming but for some clients, and on some occasions, is a worthwhile service.

Cashing up

Cashing up should be carried out at least once a day. This is the process of reconciling the cash till roll with the money actually in the till, which should of course be the same. The system of recording money taken varies from till to till but the procedure is in essence the same. Each till will have a float, a fixed amount of money which always remains in the till and is used for providing change when there is little cash in the till at the beginning of the day. The float is usually £30–£50. The total amount of cash in the till must be counted and the float removed from this total. The value of cheques should be counted, as should credit and debit card transactions if these are recorded on the till roll. Each total should be the same as is recorded on the till roll. If the totals do not match there could be a number of reasons:

◆ incorrect additions
◆ incorrect recording in the till
◆ wrong change given.

Whatever the reason the figures will need to be checked until a balance is reached. This can take time and highlights the need for accuracy at the time of the transaction.

Banking

Banking is often the responsibility of a member of the admin. staff, who checks the cash, cheques and card receipts before completing the necessary banking details on the forms provided by the bank. Money is usually banked twice a week depending on the amounts of cash taken. A bank book must be kept which records all money taken and the amount of each banking. These figures are reconciled with the bank statements received each month, which record all money banked by the practice as well as the money spent.

Accounts

In mixed practices farming clients normally receive monthly accounts. These accounts list all work carried out by the practice during the previous month, the charges made and the VAT. Many practices also add a prompt payment discount to the client's account, which is deducted if the account is paid by a certain date.

Bad debts

By asking clients to pay their bills at the time of treatment, bad debts should be avoided. This is the theory but, in practice, as support staff know this system is by no means foolproof. In Chapter 3 we discussed the many reasons clients give for not paying their bills at the time and some of the measures which can be used to encourage payment. However if all else fails the practice needs a credit control system to recover bad debts. The commonest credit control systems used are credit-control agencies, solicitors and in-house credit control.

The use of credit-control agencies is quite common and the results can be successful. The agency provides a series of standard letters for the debt controller in the practice to send to clients. The first letter is normally from the practice, reminding the client that the bill is still not paid and that if payment is not received by a certain date the debt will be placed in the hands of a debt-collecting agency. It is usually this letter that produces the most success as many clients do not want their financial details to be handed on to a debt-collecting agency for fear of a future bad credit rating. If payment is not received on this letter, the agency takes over and sends a series of letters, the final one stating that legal proceedings are about to commence. The agency will then use their solicitor to try to recover the debt through the courts. Veterinary practices normally pay a fixed fee to the agency for each client they send for debt recovery, although some agencies charge a percentage of the debt recovered.

Bad debts can be handled by the practice solicitors who, like the debt-collecting agency, will write to the client for debt recovery and then take legal action if the debt is not paid. Solicitors' fees for this service vary but can be expensive.

Bad debt recovery can be handled entirely in-house. The person responsible for credit control will write letters to the clients requesting payment and, if this is not forthcoming, inform clients that the practice will take them to the Small Claims Court. This can be a lengthy procedure and involves much form filling, but it is straightforward and cheaper than using either the debt-collecting agency or a solicitor.

Recovering bad debts is time consuming, costly and not very successful. Whichever system is used, success depends on bad debts being dealt with quickly and not left for weeks or months before they are addressed. The quicker the debtor is contacted the quicker or more likely the debt will be paid. Bad debtors often know the legal system off by heart and can delay proceedings, make counter claims and then offer to pay a £100 debt at £1 a month. The message is – avoid bad debts, be vigilant about asking people to pay at the time and don't let a potential bad debt accumulate. It is the role of the debt controller to monitor the debtor's list on a regular basis and take action early on unpaid invoices.

Petty cash

All veterinary practices have petty cash which can be used to purchase small items for cash, such as food, camera films, or reimbursement for petrol. The petty cash book is used to record every cash payment and allocate it to a purchase code so that accurate accounts can be kept by the book-keeper. A fixed amount of petty cash will be available each month, say £500. At the end of each month the cash spent will be totalled in the petty cash book and a cheque (called an imprest cheque) is written for that amount, and cashed at the bank from the practice bank account. The cash is placed back in the petty cash box so that the cash total is brought back to the fixed monthly amount.

Figure 12   Petty Cash Book

		£ Expenditure	Balance
			500.00
2.3.01	petrol	26.00	474.00
6.3.01	stamps	10.50	463.50
10.3.01	petrol	24.00	439.50
	films	12.00	
20.3.01	cleaning materials	10.00	417.50
28.3.01	coffee	3.50	414.00
TOTAL		86.00	414.00

Money remaining   £414.00

\+   +

imprest cheque   £86.00

↓   ↓

restored petty cash balance   **£500.00**

Spending the money

Purchasing goods

Some members of support staff will have responsibility for purchasing goods, these may be drugs, equipment or office items such as stationary. Goods are purchased through wholesalers or direct from veterinary companies and manufacturers.

Wholesalers

The majority of drugs are purchased from wholesalers who provide a variety of methods and equipment for drug ordering. Orders may be telephoned, faxed or emailed through to the wholesaler, who will then generally ring, fax or email back to the practice with confirmation of the order and details of any drugs which are not available and have been put on back order. This means that they will be delivered as soon as they are available.

Veterinary companies and manufacturers

Drug and equipment orders may be made direct to manufacturers with whom the practice has an account. This may involve telephoning, faxing or posting order forms to the company.

The purchasing of goods is a responsible task and normally the purchase of goods must be authorised or purchased by a named person in the practice. Purchase orders are forms which detail the items ordered and are signed by an authorised person in the practice. They usually carry a unique order number by which the purchase order form can always be identified. If the practice does not operate a purchase order system, suppliers will often request orders for goods to be sent on practice headed notepaper simply to prove the authenticity of the order.

The person responsible for purchasing is not always the person responsible for paying for them. Many practices will have a member of the admin. section whose role is to pay all invoices and accounts. This role is often associated with the book-keeper in the practice. Payment for goods may be on account, on invoice, money sent with order or by credit card.

Accounts

If the practice has an account with a supplier the goods may be ordered without payment and an account will be sent to the practice, normally on a monthly basis.

Invoices

Invoices for goods purchased are normally sent within a week or ten days and will have an expected pay-by date on the invoice, or a request to pay within a set number of days. Payment of invoices is at the discretion of the practice but generally they are not paid until the pay-by date. Payment may be by cheque signed by the authorised signatories or by computerised bank transfers, where money is transferred from the practice account to the supplier's account electronically.

Money sent with order

If the practice does not have an account with a supplier they may be asked to send the money (in the form of a cheque) with the order. The disadvantages of this system are that the company has to receive the money before the goods are dispatched and this can take a number of days. More seriously, the money is paid immediately rather than two or three weeks after the goods have been received and if the goods have to be returned credit notes or reimbursements have to be organised.

Credit cards

This method of payment is becoming more common for purchasing items. However access to, and use of, the credit card has to be limited to named users to prevent overspending and abuse. Goods can be purchased using the card either over the telephone or by presentation of the card by the authorised signatory.

Stock control

Stock control goes hand in hand with practice finance. Good stock control is about saving the practice money. Money should not be tied up in drugs sitting on shelves not being used, or reaching their expiry dates, when it could be used to pay bills or earn interest. There must be good control over all items purchased but the most important area is that of drug purchase.

Some veterinary practices have computerised stock control where all items purchased are keyed into the computer, and each time a drug is dispensed the amount is automatically recorded by the computer from the client record. Every item will have maximum and minimum stock levels so the computer can

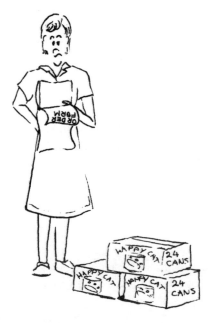
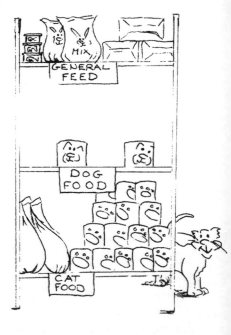

generate stock reports listing those drugs and the quantities which need to be reordered. Manual stock control depends on careful monitoring of stock on shelves and a very good knowledge of drug usage.

Many wholesalers now provide an aid to manual stock control in the form of hand-held equipment listing all the drugs held by the practice and the stock levels required. The stock controller then simply keys into the equipment the amount of each drug on the shelf and a drug order can be generated for all items which need to be restocked. This order is then passed to the wholesaler by electronic transfer.

Stock rotation is a vital part of good stock control, when new drugs arrive they should always be placed behind the existing drugs on the shelves so that the drug with the earlier expiry date is used first.

Here are the main principles of good stock control.

⇨ Maintain minimum stock levels at all times.

⇨ Only order items when they are needed, do not stock pile.

⇨ Use consistent stock rotation.

⇨ Aim to stock the financial equivalent of no more than three weeks worth of stock. So, if the practice normally spends £40,000 per month on drug, then ideally no more than £30,000 worth of drugs should be in the practice as stock.

Paying the money

Someone has to pay the staff and this role usually falls to one of the office administrators or a practice manager. There are a number of ways salaries can be paid:

◆ weekly

◆ monthly

◆ cash

◆ cheque

◆ bank credit transfer. In this way, money is paid directly from the practice bank account into an employee's bank account.

As well as a basic salary some practices provide what are called fringe benefits such as:

◆ private health insurance

◆ pension scheme

◆ car

◆ accommodation

◆ telephone

◆ uniform.

Income tax must be paid on salaries received and also on fringe benefits. An employee's taxable income is the income on which they are taxed, after all tax allowances have been made. Veterinary practices operate the PAYE (pay as you earn) scheme, so all employees are subject to taxation at source, i.e. tax is removed from their salary at the time it is paid. Tax rates and tax codes are subject to variation depending on government policy.

Annual tax bands

These are the different tax bands on which tax is paid and are set each year by the government at budget time.

Figure 13   Tax rates

Tax	For year 2000–01	£ taxable pay Budget proposals for year 2001–02
10%	up to £1,520	up to £1,880
22%	from £1,521–£28,400	from £1,880–£29,400
40%	from £28,401 upwards	from £29,401 upwards

Tax codes

All employees are allocated a personal tax code which reflects their financial circumstances; whether they are single or married and if they have dependants. The tax code gives the person's allowable non-taxable income. So, for example, someone with a tax code of 438L (the tax code for a single person with no dependants) will be allowed to earn £4,380 before they start paying tax.

If we take an example of someone earning £10,000 per annum with a tax code of 438L their taxable income would be calculated as follows.

£10,000 – £4,380 = £5,620 taxable income

10% tax paid on	£1,520		=	£152
22% tax paid on	£4,100	(£5,620 – £1,520)	=	£902
Total tax bill			=	£1,054

National insurance

Employees must also pay National Insurance (NI) contributions which go towards contributory benefits: retirement pension, incapacity benefit and unemployment benefit. Most employees pay Class 1 National Insurance which is made up of an employee's and an employer's share. The employee's share is deducted from their salary while the employer's share is paid separately by the employer.

National Insurance contributions are worked out on the employee's gross pay before any tax has been removed. The lower earnings limit for paying National Insurance is currently £67 per week; if the employee earns less than this they pay no NI. NI is paid on a sliding scale, the more you earn the more you pay. Everyone has a NI number given to them by the Department of Social Security Contributions Agency, the number consists of two letters, six numbers and one letter, in the format AB 23 48 76 C.

Pay slips

Many veterinary practices now use computer programmes such as Sage Payroll to calculate staff salaries and to generate pay slips. This saves a large amount of time in calculating tax and NI from the tables provided by the tax office. The form of a wages slip varies but all contain the following information:

NI number
Tax code
Employee name
Date
Tax month
Type of payment (weekly/monthly)
Payments: salary
            overtime
            sick pay
            maternity pay
Deductions: PAYE
            NI
            Pension.

There are two types of form associated with salary which most employees will receive during their employment.

At the end of each financial year employees' total salary, tax and NI contributions are calculated and employees are given a P60 form which lists all this information. Duplicate P14 forms are sent by the employer to the tax office.

When an employee leaves their job, they are given a P45 form by their employer which states all pay, tax and NI received and paid by the employee during the current tax year. This form must be presented to a new employer so that the correct tax and NI can be deducted when the employee starts their new job.

Statutory sick pay (SSP) and statutory maternity pay (SMP) are paid to employees who are sick or become pregnant so long as the required conditions for payment are met. SSP is currently paid to sick employees who are away from work for more than three qualifying days. At the moment, SMP is paid to pregnant employees for 18 weeks.

Staff salaries form a major part of a veterinary practice expenditure and the payroll administrator's job is a responsible one. Salaries must be paid correctly, overtime and statutory payments, tax and NI calculated accurately and payments must be made on time.

Managing the money

This role normally falls to senior administrators or practice managers, but it is important that all staff understand the basics of money management in veterinary practice, so that they are aware of the need to make a profit, pay the bills, practice stock control and avoid waste.

Income and expenditure

Income is the money received by the practice from the sale of goods and services. Expenditure is the money spent by the practice on the goods and services it requires to operate. Expenditure is made up from following two areas.

1 Expenses – the constant things which the practice has to spend money on in order to carry out its business, such as rent, rates, electricity, telephone and salaries. These are called fixed costs because they stay the same regardless of the profit or loss the practice may make or how much business there is.

2 Purchases – the items which the practice has to buy in order that it can provide and sell its services, such as drugs and equipment. These are called variable costs and change according to how much work the practice does.

Income must exceed expenditure if the practice is to make a profit. For example:

Income £10,000 – Expenditure £8,000   =   Profit £2,000

Income £10,000 – Expenditure £11,000   =   Loss £1,000

It is important to understand that income is not the same as profit. When a client buys a bag of dog food, the profit the practice makes is the difference between the price they paid for it and the price they charged the client.

As well as the money made in profit, the practice is likely to have financial assets called current assets, such as:

buildings
cars
equipment
money invested
stock held by the practice: e.g. drugs
debtors – the people who owe the practice money.

They may also have financial liabilities called current liabilities such as:
overdraft
bank loan
mortgage.

Current assets – Current liabilities   =   Working capital

Working capital is the money actually available to the owners to spend on running the business.

The person managing the money must produce several financial reports each month in order to keep abreast of the financial situation of the practice. The two main reports are the profit and loss account and the balance sheet. The profit and loss account should be produced monthly and is simply the balance between the costs of running the practice and the income of the practice in the current financial year. The balance sheet is produced at less frequent intervals and is in effect a snapshot of the worth of the veterinary practice at a given moment in time.

Summary

- Receptionists in particular are responsible for handling money paid by clients, and cashing up and reconciling the till.
- Staff taking money need to be able to generate invoices and receipts, accept money in the form of cash, cheques and credit and debit cards and be able to calculate VAT.
- Bad debts may be handled by the veterinary practice, a debt collecting agency or by the practice solicitors.
- Drugs are one of a veterinary practice's biggest expenditures and stock control is a vital part of managing money. Minimum stock levels and stock rotation are the most important aspects of good stock control.
- The purchase of goods by the practice may be on account, on invoice, money sent with order or by credit card.
- Staff salaries are paid weekly or monthly in cash, by cheque or bank credit transfer.
- Income tax must be paid on all taxable salary and fringe benefits; tax codes and tax rates are set by the government each year.
- NI contributions must be paid by all employees currently earning over £67 per week – they pay for retirement pensions, incapacity benefit and unemployment benefit.
- Practice income must exceed expenditure for the practice to make a profit.

- All businesses have financial assets and financial liabilities and the difference between these two is the working capital.
- The profit and loss account and the balance sheet are the two most important financial reports needed to assess how the veterinary practice is functioning as a business.

What support staff say

Q: What part do you play in taking money, spending money or dealing with money in the practice?

Christine: 'I deal with client payments, cash up, am responsible for petty cash and chase bad debtors'

Denise: 'I order stock and drugs and take money from clients when I work on the reception desk'

April: 'I am responsible for doing the practice accounts and I deal with the bad debtors'

Margaret: 'I deal with money indirectly by making sure insurance claims are sent in quickly and filled out correctly. I will follow up any problems there may be with the insurance company. I also negotiate with the various animal charities regarding help for some of our clients and am the charities liaison officer for the practice. I get a great deal of satisfaction from being able to help some of our clients who have difficulty paying their bills and at the same time I am helping the practice by making sure our work is paid for.'

Elaine: 'I deal with client invoices at reception and balance the cash at the end of the day . I send bi-monthly accounts and monitor for bad debtors to ensure these are kept to a minimum, I also monitor instalment accounts to make sure they are up to date.'

Liz: 'I spend the practice money on drugs and equipment and when I work in the dispensary I take money from clients for drugs. I have to check wholesalers' invoices against drugs received and I am responsible for the stock control of our drugs'

Exercise 5

Look at the different ways clients pay their bills, e.g. cash, cheque debit and credit card and try to assess what percentage of clients pay in each of these different ways.

Find out how your practice deals with bad debtors and try to work out the percentage of bad debts which are recovered by the system the practice has in place.

Find out the current values for the tax rate bands, personal allowances and the lower earnings limit of National Insurance and the extent of Statutory Maternity Pay, mentioned on pages 60–61.

6

Support staff and the office

Many veterinary support staff have an administrative role behind the scenes. They rarely deal with clients but they do deal with manufacturers, suppliers, wholesalers and servicing and maintenance companies. They have an important role to play because the other veterinary support staff would have difficulty carrying out their roles without those who give administrative support. Ordering drugs, equipment supplies, ensuring well-maintained equipment, computer troubleshooting and organising the mail are just a few of the vital processes.

In larger practices there is often a member of support staff who takes on the role of office manager and is responsible for the daily running of the office and its staff. In smaller practices office tasks such as filing, dealing with in-coming and out-going mail, word processing and office stock control, are allocated to different members of staff as part of their overall responsibilities. For example, a nurse may also have responsibility for filing client x-rays or lab reports, a receptionist may spend some of her time word processing, producing veterinary reports, letters or perhaps display or publicity material.

Office and administrative tasks vary a great deal and require as much care and accuracy as any of the other jobs in the veterinary practice.

The mail

Someone has to sort through the pile of letters which arrives each morning at the veterinary surgery. This role often falls to a practice manager but, in the absence of a practice manager, the role is often allocated to a member of support staff.

Incoming mail falls into a number of broad categories:

◆ personal letters
◆ lab reports

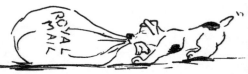

- invoices from veterinary suppliers
- cheques from clients paying their accounts
- journals and magazines
- advertising leaflets.

Mail needs to be sorted and distributed, priority letters identified and manufacturers' information passed to the correct people in the practice. So it is often helpful if there is system of trays or pigeon holes for vets' and nurses' mail.

Mail also leaves the practice on a daily basis in the form of letters, accounts, cheques to veterinary suppliers, equipment orders, laboratory material for analysis and parcels. The person responsible for the mail should ensure addresses and return addresses are clear and legible and apply the correct postage to letters and parcels. It helps if there is a box for first and a box for second class mail so that the urgency of the letters is clear.

Some practices have franking machines which frank all mail with first and second class dated franking stamps as well as the practice logo if required. Franked mail is then placed in special Post Office bags and either delivered to the Post Office or collected by the postman. Franking machines are usually rented and have to be kept in credit by electronic transfer of funds from the practice bank account. It also costs money for the post to be collected each day from the veterinary practice. However in large, busy practices franking machines and mail collection save considerably on staff time and can be a great convenience.

Parcels, especially those containing veterinary samples, must be correctly and carefully wrapped and if a franking system is used, weighed and the weight checked against Post Office parcel charges, so that the correct postage can be generated by the franking machine.

Filing

Even in the computer age there is still manual filing to be carried out, for example:

◆ lab reports
◆ client letters
◆ x-rays
◆ invoices
◆ client records (for the non-computerised practices).

Physical filing systems vary from simple card indexes to automatic computer filing. The commonest non-computerised systems used are A-Z folders in filing cabinets for letters, the Carter Parrat system for filing client record cards and box files for storing and filing x-rays.

The practice's largest filing system is of course for its clients' records and the ideal method is to use a computer. There are a number of alternative ways to file documents in manual systems. Let's look for example at the different ways a lab report could be filed:

Lab report number	2466
Date	21-7-00
Animal	Bob
Animal record number	44667
Species	Dog
Owner	Mrs S Brown
Address	25 Old Street, New Town

Do you file the lab report by:

◆ lab report number?
◆ date?
◆ species of animal?
◆ animal record number?
◆ name of owner?

Each practice will have their own preferences for filing, depending on the way they may need to retrieve the record in the future, the important thing is to follow this preference and be consistent.

Filing requires great care, one mis-filed document can result in hours of searching and, as we all know, it is always the file you need which is the one that you can't find! If Bob's lab report should be filed by lab report number but has actually been filed by animal record number there are a lot of records to be sorted through before the report is found.

Practice forms

All practices seem to generate large numbers of forms for the many procedures they carry out. Someone has to be responsible for the form bank, filing master copies and photocopying forms when required. Forms need to be consistent and use the same type style, practice logo and colouring if they are to look professional. This is a job for someone with an eye for detail and design.

Stationery

How many pens, elastic bands, paper clips and appointment cards fall out of the stationery cupboard in your practice when the door is opened? Or is everything neatly stacked and labelled? The answer depends on the efficiency of the member of staff responsible for ordering and organising the stationery.

This is the person whose job it is to look through the wonderful world of the stationery catalogue and decide which is the best buy in black biros or marker pens. Or whether buying packs of twenty A4 files at £15 and keeping ten on the shelves is cheaper than buying only ten files at £1.50 each for immediate use. Stationery catalogues are like Aladdin's cave, full of tempting jewels which 'you simply cannot do without'. So the stationery buyer has to exert great control over the needs and wants of the staff in the practice. Printed stationery, such as headed notepaper, will be ordered through a printer but competitive prices will still have to be negotiated.

Whoever is responsible for stationery ordering must practice good stock control, monitoring levels and ordering only when stock is getting low. At the same time they may need to remember future plans, so that if a new vet is to be added to the notepaper in a month's time, the printer should be told before the next six months' worth of notepaper is printed.

Pens have a magical ability to disappear in their hundreds in veterinary practices – although practices receive so many free pens from veterinary companies, there always seems to be a pen shortage. One member of support staff I know, who is responsible for stationery ordering, tried refusing to issue anyone with a new pen unless they presented her with the old empty one. As you might expect the experiment did not last long! This may have been carrying things a little too far, but raiding lab coat pockets and cars on a regular basis can be very productive. Also requesting that everyone bring in at least six of their spare pens every month can increase pen stocks dramatically. The point is that stationery should not be seen as available in large quantities to all. Some control over its issue and use is essential to avoid wastage. Why buy large post-it notes if smaller ones will do? Try supplying telephone message pads to prevent messages being written on more expensive notepaper, or worse, appointment cards.

Secretarial services

A large amount of secretarial work and word processing is carried out in many practices, especially in practices where reports have to be produced for referred or large animal work. Full-time secretaries or support staff

who also have other duties may have this role and be responsible for:
- client letters
- veterinary reports
- internal forms
- practice documents
- newsletters
- client leaflets.

More and more in-house and desk-top publishing is being carried out in veterinary practices. Packages like PageMaker, Publisher and Quark Express enable the production of in-house client and staff newsletters and professional-looking leaflets and handouts. It may be that staff require external training for this kind of word processing, but it can be well worth while and the results can be impressive.

It is very important that any promotional and client material looks professional. Clients are far more critical than they used to be and more used to seeing professionally produced literature. Well-designed and produced handouts show the client that the practice is professional and organised, badly photocopied handouts suggest that the practice does not care about its image or the work it does.

Office equipment

Gone are the days when there was a telephone, a Gestetner machine for duplicating and a guillotine. There is now an impressive array of office equipment in most veterinary practices for example:
- photocopiers
- printers
- fax machines
- franking machines
- multi-line telephone systems
- computers and personal computers (PCs)
- electronic scales
- shredding machines.

Support staff need not only to know how to use this equipment, but also how to carry out basic trouble-shooting and be aware of health and safety when using them.

Staff may have to operate multi-line telephone systems, so that they can re-direct and retrieve calls, use paging systems and voice calls and re-direct phones to night duty vets.

Photocopiers are becoming more sophisticated and staff must be able to produce copies of a range of documents of the appropriate size and colour of paper, single-sided and double-sided, as well as knowing how to unjam paper from the rollers and change the toner when it is empty.

Franking machine use requires knowledge of how to refill with money, set correct dates and apply correct postage to parcels and letters.

Whenever any of this office equipment is used, staff must know how to carry out general safety checks for frayed wires, blackened sockets or damage to the equipment, and report problems to the health and safety officer or their supervisor. They also require a basic understanding of how the equipment works so that they can identify problems and have some idea of how to solve them. Simple equipment maintenance and being able to reset dates, telephone numbers, change toners, printer ribbons and so on are all part of the job.

Computers

Computers have revolutionised the administrative work in veterinary practices. There are still practices which do not have computerised client records or accounts, but in many practices computers are now used for all or many of the following procedures:

- maintaining client records and accounts
- practice book-keeping and accounting
- PAYE and employee salaries
- data retrieval and reports
- word processing
- email, websites and internet
- stock control.

There are three main aspects to consider when it comes to understanding the use and how to use computers in veterinary practice.

1 Specific Software

Every veterinary practice which is computerised uses specialised software. These packages will vary in detail but in essence all provide the ability to produce and maintain the following material.

Client records

This will contain details of client's name, address and telephone number, animal's name and record number as well as the pet's age, species, sex and colour, vaccination details, insurance details, micro-chipping. Details of all treatment and drugs prescribed will be recorded and stored on the computer.

Client invoices

The computer can be set to produce client invoices at the time of treatment as well as monthly invoices for account holders.

Data retrieval

From the information on the client's record all kinds of data can be produced for practice planning, marketing strategies and management information.

Vaccination reminders

Vaccination reminders for each month can be generated from client computer records.

Drug labelling

As the consultation details and drugs prescribed are keyed into the client record by the vet or nurse a drug label can be generated with all the required dispensing details.

Stock control

The computer can also be used to set drug stock levels. As dispensed drugs are recorded the computer will alter stock records and highlight low stock levels and drugs which need reordering.

Everyone new to veterinary practice will require training on these individual systems because most are adapted to the specific needs of the practice. Training may be in-house by other members of staff or in training sessions provided by the veterinary computer company trainers.

2 Standard Software

Many veterinary practices will use standardised 'off the shelf' computer software, often part of the Microsoft Office suite to carry out a variety of tasks.

Word processing

The production of letters, reports and leaflets using a PC, which may or may not be connected to other PCs in the practice.

Spreadsheets

These can be tabulated reports, financial or other information which is best displayed and understood by presenting it in the form of a large table of data. Information on spreadsheets can be varied and altered, and the effect of changes in figures or formulae will be automatically registered on the spreadsheet. Spreadsheets are useful tools for planning and estimating budgets.

Desk top publishing (DTP)

Using special publishing packages, very professional-looking illustrated colour documents, newsletters and pamphlets can be produced in-house. These packages are ideal for the production of client newsletters and display material.

Practice accounting

Accounting packages like Sage allow all the practice book-keeping to be computerised saving an enormous amount of time.

PAYE

These packages enable all employees' salaries to be calculated, tax and National Insurance to be calculated and deducted, and full PAYE records to be kept on the computer. The same packages enable the generation of salary slips.

Salary payment and invoice payment

Several bank packages allow for the direct payment of money from the practice bank account into other bank accounts. This enables salaries to be paid directly from the practice account into the employees' bank accounts and invoices paid directly to suppliers' bank accounts. Money can also be transferred between different practice accounts to allow for an efficient cash flow.

Email, websites and the internet

Email clients allow access to emailing and the internet, while a variety of customised packages are now available for practices to produce and maintain their own websites. Alternatively the practice may commission a website company to design and maintain a website for them.

Training packages

There is a considerable amount of training available on CD Roms and increasingly on the internet.

Familiarity with standard office programmes will enable support staff to use these bought-in packages without further training. For support staff new to such software training will be required either in-house from other members of staff or via the many widely available computer courses.

The hardware and mechanics

As computer systems improve we all have less need to know what goes on 'underneath the bonnet' of the computer. It is still however extremely useful to have a basic knowledge of how to respond to such events as error messages. Also to be able to check connections, change faulty printers and keyboards, back up the system and avoid possibly one of the major causes of computer problems by shutting down the computer system correctly.

There may be someone in the practice whose role it is to act as a trouble shooter when there is a computer problem. But it is still important that support staff have enough knowledge of the computer and computer language if only so that they can talk to the computer help line, answer questions about the problem and understand the advice given to them.

Data protection

Veterinary practices now often hold a considerable amount of information about clients and their pets on the practice computer, such as names and addresses, telephone numbers, money owed, bad debts incurred. Like all other businesses holding this kind of computerised information, veterinary practices must comply with the Data Protection Act which protects the personal rights of individuals. The Data Protection Act is dealt with in more detail in Chapter 8.

Health and safety

An awareness of, and compliance with, health and safety should run through everything support staff do in the veterinary practice.

The owner of the practice, as the employer, has a legal duty under the Health and Safety at Work Act to produce a practice Health and Safety Policy committing the practice to achieving good standards of health and safety. They must also ensure as far as is reasonably practicable the health and safety of all their employees, and they must train their employees in all aspects of health and safety which affect the work they do.

Employees in turn also have legal duties regarding health and safety. They must take reasonable care of their own health and safety, follow all the health and safety procedures of the practice and undertake all the practice health and safety training. It is also part of their responsibility to inform their employer of any potentially unsafe working conditions. The organisation responsible for monitoring health and safety in the workplace is the Health and Safety Executive (HSE) which has considerable powers and can shut a business down completely if there is a major health and safety risk.

Support staff should be aware of the health and safety measures the veterinary practice takes to protect them. In some practices support staff are actively involved in administering the health and safety policy, helping to carry out risk assessments and acting as first aiders and fire officers.

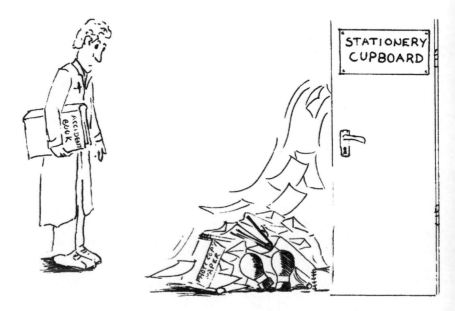

Many of the health and safety activities of the practice are associated with assessing the risk to employees of using potentially hazardous substances or carrying out potentially hazardous tasks. This process is called risk assessment.

Risk assessment

Risk assessments identify hazards, assess risks and decide what control measures are needed for safe working. So what do we mean by hazard and risk?

A hazard is something which has the potential to cause harm – a motor car for example. A risk is the likelihood of the harm actually occurring – the motor car hitting a pedestrian.

In the veterinary practice, x-raying a dog would be considered a potential hazard because of the radiation staff would be exposed to. The actual risk is the likelihood of staff actually being exposed to the radiation. Because radiation is hazardous, control measures are put in place which reduce the risk as much as possible, including the wearing of lead aprons and gloves, staying outside the x-ray room or area when x-raying is taking place, no staff under the age of 18 being allowed to help with x-raying. Every veterinary practice will have the Local Rules to provide guidance on x-ray procedures.

To ensure a safe workplace a number of risk assessments have by law to be carried out by all employers looking at possible or known hazards, what the risks are to staff and what control measures must be put in place. These risk assessments must be carried out in the following areas in veterinary practice:

- general health and safety in the workplace
- electrical safety
- manual handling
- display screen equipment
- young people at work
- lone workers
- personal protective equipment
- new and expectant mothers
- fire
- first aid
- ionising radiation
- control of substances hazardous to health (COSHH).

All these assessments affect support staff in some way, whether it is the receptionist left to 'man' the reception desk alone at lunchtimes, the secretary who spends much of her day working on a word processor, the nurse helping to x-ray animals or the member of staff dispensing drugs to clients.

The named person in the practice responsible for carrying out health and safety is often the practice manager and it is to them that support staff should report any worries they have about their own or others' safety.

For any activity for which a risk has been identified there should be a practice Standard Operating Procedure (SOP), a simple document which sets out how the activity should be safely carried out, so that there is as little risk as possible to the member of staff involved.

All staff should be aware of the SOPs which affect them and follow all the instructions given. SOPs are especially important when dealing with hazardous substances, and staff must be sure they know how to handle those drugs which have been identified as having a risk attached to their use. Support staff should also know what the procedure is if they spill a drug or accidentally inject themselves, and be sure they will be able to identify whether the drug is hazardous, how they will clear up the spillage, and if they should seek medical advice about injecting the drug into themselves.

In accordance with the Health and Safety (First Aid) Regulations 1981 practices should have a named person responsible for overseeing the provision of first aid in the practice. The practice should have available a First Aid Box containing suitable first aid materials to be used if a member of staff requires first aid attention due to an accident. If the practice employs more than 20 people it should also appoint a member of staff as the qualified first aider. Normally a practice will send an interested member of staff on an approved First Aid course (run by St John's Ambulance or Red Cross).

All accidents at work, however small, should be reported in the Accident Book, giving details of date, when, where and how the accident happened and what treatment was given. Serious accidents and incidents, or diseases contracted through the work the employee does, should also be reported to the Health and Safety Executive under a regulation called the Reporting of Incidents, Diseases and Dangerous Occurrences (RIDDOR). This reporting responsibility lies with the appointed health and safety officer of the practice.

All staff should be familiar with the practice fire regulations and know what to do in the event of a fire, where the fire exits are and where the fire assembly point is. Regular fire drills should be carried out in the practice so that staff are familiar with fire escapes and building evacuation procedures.

The veterinary practice should always be monitoring and reviewing health and safety. Things change, new equipment may be bought, new procedures introduced, and different drugs used. All these changes mean health and safety has to be reassessed, and support staff have a real responsibility and part to play in looking at how such changes affect practice health and safety, not just to protect themselves but also their colleagues.

Summary

- Office administration is an important support staff role in veterinary practice.
- Administration tasks include filing, organising mail, stock control, stationery supplies, secretarial work and the use of office equipment.
- Many areas of veterinary practice are now computerised and most support staff will be involved in using computer systems.
- Veterinary practices have both specialist and standard computer software, the former requires specialist staff training while the latter is common to many other businesses.
- Health and safety pervades all aspects of work in veterinary practice.
- Risk assessments are undertaken to assess the potential hazard and risks of substances used and activities carried out by employees.
- Support staff should be aware of the health and safety aspects of their work and comply with all the practice health and safety policies and procedures.

What support staff say

Q: How do you use the computer in your job?

Pat: 'I access client case notes, produce invoices, add new clients to the data base and use the computer to obtain information about clients' animals so that we can send promotional literature to selected clients.'

April: 'I do the practice book-keeping using a computer accounting package and I also use the computer to do all the staff salaries.'

Elaine: 'I use the computer to book client appointments, enter lab results, produce invoices, maintain client records and send recalls for vaccinations. I also liaise with our computer company over computer problems and queries.'

Margaret: 'It's my job to be the trouble-shooter for computer problems. I can sort out many of the basic problems which arise and enjoy finding out about the extra information the computer can be used to provide.'

Liz: 'I use the computer for stock control, and producing reports on drug sales and trends. I also process the drug orders via the internet. I use the PC to write letters and create spreadsheets.'

Q: What office work are you regularly involved with?

Pat: 'Photocopying, faxing and making sure we always have enough leaflets to give to clients.'

Elaine: 'I have to organise reception staff rotas and I liaise with vets so that I know when they are on holiday so that 'named vet' appointments are not booked when they are away. I run the VAT book and monthly accounts printouts for the practice manager. When we have promotions I generate the targeted client lists so that marketing information and invitations can be sent to clients.'

Christine: 'I file lab reports and x-rays.'

April: 'I order stationery, file paperwork, do lots of word processing and deal with veterinary suppliers.'

Liz: 'I order stationery, write up and file lab reports, use the fax machine and deal with the mail.'

Exercise 6

List the office and administrative tasks you carry out, and work out the time you spend each day on each task compared with dealing with clients.

Read your practice Health and Safety Policy; who is the person responsible for Health and Safety in the practice? List the measures the practice has taken to ensure you are safe while carrying out your job.

7

How support staff contribute to sales and marketing

The first question many support staff ask when sales and marketing is mentioned is, 'what's the difference?' The answer is 'rather a lot'.

Sales or selling is the promotion of our services and veterinary products which results in the client purchasing those services or products.

Marketing is the process of matching the practice services and products to the clients' needs and promoting them in order to build a long term and profitable relationship between the business and the client. Put more simply it is finding out what the client wants and giving it to them

The veterinary market is changing all the time, clients are becoming more demanding, but are also prepared to spend more money on good services. Ten or fifteen years ago the veterinary practice simply cured sick pets, and apart from a few wormers or flea powders nothing else was sold to the client. The practice most certainly did not advertise its existence and selling was not seen as a role for veterinary staff. Indeed until only a couple of years ago the RCVS frowned upon any kind of advertising by veterinary practices, considering it to be unprofessional.

Well, things have changed. There is more and more competition for veterinary practices not only from other practices and chains of practices, but also from pet superstores and, increasingly, websites selling pet products and providing veterinary information.

The veterinary practice which does not boost its income from pet product sales, or actively market itself to the public, will be struggling to survive over the next 5–10 years.

It has never been so important for all the staff in the veterinary practice to be aware of the importance of good sales and marketing techniques.

What is selling

Selling until recently has been a controversial issue for many veterinary surgeons. They have found it difficult to reconcile the perceived 'pushy' image of the sales person with the clinical care of animals. But the money from sales is now an important part of veterinary income and the image of selling has changed.

Selling in veterinary practice is now considered professional. It helps clients make informed decisions about the health care product that is best for their pet. It is far better for them to purchase goods from a veterinary practice where they can get expert advice, than from a pet superstore where the products are simply piled high on the shelves and they have to make their choice unaided.

Selling is no longer considered unethical. Practices are not selling useless or unnecessary products to clients, but beneficial and reliable goods which often form part of a health care programme for, say, weight control or dental hygiene.

All veterinary practices need to look at pet care from the client's point of view. The 'one stop shop' is becoming more popular for busy working clients. They are pleased to be able to take Bonzo for his booster and at the same time purchase his year's worth of flea control, wormers, a new doggy duvet, a large bag of dog food which will last him for the next month and the impulse purchase of the squeezy toy because Bonzo has been left on his own all today.

By providing quality health care products as well as giving professional advice and care the practice is giving added value to the client and increases the chances of bonding them to the practice, thus securing a regular customer who recommends the practice to their friends.

The main benefits of good sales in veterinary practice are:

♦ increase in practice income

- increase in opportunities to bond clients to the practice
- part of a total health care service for the client
- make efficient and effective use of waiting room space.

The role of support staff in selling

Support staff are crucial to veterinary practice sales. They are the front line for selling products and services to clients and are generally responsible for the majority of selling in the practice. Consequently they need to have a very good understanding of the art and science of selling and look upon selling as a skill, not just something extra that they do when they have finished making appointments and answering the telephone.

These are some of the basic steps to successful selling.

▷ Talk to the client, identify their needs and wants through careful questioning and listening.

▷ Offer appropriate products for the client's needs and talk to them about the products, their use and benefits.

▷ Know the major benefits and features of the products for sale, if it is for example, a dried dog food, know:

> the ingredients
> the costs of a day's feed
> the other brands and what the key differences are
> the age range it is intended for
> how palatable it is
> that the client can have a refund if their pet doesn't like the taste.

▷ It is always a selling point if the staff member can tell the client that they use the product for their own pet, but only of course if they really do!

▷ Look for opportunities to sell/recommend products. For example, after a pet has had a dental, offer the client dental care products such as toothpaste and brushes or rasks. After a first vaccination of a new puppy offer bedding and toys, and give information on changing from puppy to adult diets.

▷ Allow the client to touch, examine or smell the products before they purchase.

▷ Display the products in an attractive way – a science all of its own. Display new products on the left-hand side of the display area as clients always look to the left of a product display first. Centre shelves always sell the most goods as they are usually at eye level, so place high-to-medium price goods in this position.

▷ Always keep the shelves well stocked, half-empty shelves put clients off buying the products.

⮑ Display products where the clients can easily see and touch them, don't have them in an inaccessible corner or behind the reception desk.

⮑ Display products in high traffic areas so that clients are constantly walking past them.

⮑ Spotlights shining on displays make them look more attractive.

⮑ Good colour co-ordination makes product displays more appealing.

And finally, think of and be able to answer the five questions most clients ask before they purchase a product.

1   What is it?
2   Why should I buy it?
3   How much is it?
4   Is it useful?
5   Do I want it now?

Support staff need to help clients answer these questions:

1   *What is it?* – A complete dried diet for adult dogs.
2   *Why should I buy it?* – It is a quality product providing a palatable balanced diet which contains all the nutrients your dog requires in one food.
3   *How much is it?* – It will cost only 37½p per day.
4   *Is it useful?* – It will maintain a healthy life for your dog.
5   *Do I want it now?* –If you buy the product today, we give you £5 to use on your next purchase. This offer ends on Friday.

Client needs and wants

There is a difference between what a client may need, and what they may want, which support staff must have clear when advising on or selling any product. We all *need* shampoo to wash our hair, this is a necessary purchase. We may *want* a particular shampoo in a fancy bottle with a designer name on it, which is much more expensive. This is not a necessary purchase in the true sense of the word, but we will get great enjoyment from using the shampoo.

It is the same with clients. They *need* to buy a flea control product to ensure their pet is free from fleas – a necessary purchase. They may *want* to buy their pet a new toy – an unnecessary purchase but the client will get tremendous pleasure from watching their pet play with the toy.

When selling to clients, staff should be aware of the difference in these sales. The practice is selling to both the needs and wants of clients. The client's wants are the non-essential products, which historically vets had difficulty accepting as items they could sell. But if the client really wants a squeaky toy or a different coloured collar for their pet, then we should be happy and able to sell them these items, because we are giving them pleasure and satisfaction and an added value service.

What is marketing?

Marketing has three main aims:

1 To ensure clients stay with the practice.
2 To generate more business from existing clients.
3 To attract new clients to the practice.

The practice is marketing to the client whenever a client comes into contact with the veterinary practice in any way. It may be just by walking past the building, reading an article in the local newspaper or picking up the practice newsletter in a friend's home.

Marketing is essential to ensure the survival of the practice and is a mixture of ingredients.

◆ The service and the product being offered – what services are provided, what new products are available.
◆ The processes of the practice – how well the telephone is answered, how easy it is to make an appointment.
◆ The location of the service and product – where the veterinary practice is, how easy it is to reach and if there is a large car park.
◆ The promotion and advertising of the service and product – how are clients told of the services and products.
◆ The price of the services and products – are they value for money?
◆ The people in the practice – the staff are the greatest marketing tool the practice has.

Marketing is used by practices to ensure that clients and potential clients are aware of all the services and products available from the practice. This is done by internal marketing and external marketing of the practice.

Internal marketing

The practice is promoted by use of:

◆ the practice staff, by the way they care for clients
◆ businss cards for all staff to give to clients
◆ practice brochures
◆ practice newsletters
◆ practice information packs to new clients
◆ practice album in waiting room
◆ information about practice services, such as nurse's clinics
◆ display boards in waiting rooms promoting new products, new services or showing work behind the scenes in the practice
◆ booster reminders
◆ sympathy cards
◆ clinical handouts
◆ VIP Clubs for the most frequent use clients
◆ 'thank you' cards to clients who recommend the practice to others

- open days
- gifts given with special promotions or with puppy party packs
- websites
- target marketing, e.g. writing to all clients with pets over seven years giving information about the practice's 'older pet' clinic.

External marketing

- The signage of the practice: is it visible, attractive, welcoming?
- The practice logo, which should be on everything which leaves the practice.
- Plastic carrier bags with the practice logo on them for clients' purchases.
- The practice uniform worn by support staff which advertises the practice if the staff are out shopping in the town at lunchtime.
- Practice logo car stickers.
- Practice ambulances carrying the logo and practice name.
- Advertising in Yellow Pages.
- Articles about the practice in the local newspaper.
- Publicity about practice events on the local radio.
- Practice staff giving talks to schools and local clubs.
- Visits to the practice by local groups and school children.
- Work experience pupils.
- Vets judging pets at local shows.
- Practice vets and staff at local country events and shows.

Marketing enhances the public image of the practice, it enables clients to evaluate the quality and service of the practice and appreciate the difference in service between your practice and the others.

There are dozens of ways the practice can be marketed so that it is kept in the public eye. If the practice does not market itself, it may not attract new clients and its competitors who are marketing themselves may not only benefit from all the potential new clients but also attract existing clients away from the practice.

The role of support staff in marketing

The moment that a client walks through the door, the staff are marketing the practice to them. It may be by a welcoming smile, the ease with which they can book their appointment or the information the receptionist gives them about puppy parties. Everything the staff do that involves communicating with the client is a form of marketing and leaves an impression, good or bad, about the practice. The role of support staff in marketing therefore can be seen as very, very important.

These are some of the many ways that the support staff can help to market the practice to clients.

⇨ Providing a quality service to the client.
⇨ Showing they care about the client and their pet.
⇨ Being friendly, helpful and sympathetic to clients and their needs.
⇨ Keeping all areas of the practice clean and tidy.
⇨ Giving clients practice newsletters, leaflets and handouts.
⇨ Advising clients on pet health care and nutrition.
⇨ Talking to clients about services.
⇨ Designing good informative displays for the waiting room.
⇨ Helping the work experience pupils who will be reporting back to their family friends and school about the practice.
⇨ Putting the practice logo or address on all literature.
⇨ Helping at practice open days.
⇨ Wearing the practice uniform with pride.
⇨ Promoting the practice image outside the practice when not at work.
⇨ Always exceeding the clients' expectations.

It is important for support staff to be aware of their role in marketing their practice. Many practices now have marketing plans in which all staff are involved. Components of a typical plan are shown in the following table.

Figure 14 Marketing plan

Aims	to increase the uptake of booster vaccinations.
Objectives	to increase the uptake by five per cent in the next year.
Targets	all clients whose pets have had vaccinations in the last three years.
Strategies	mail all clients explaining the benefits of vaccination and offer 10% off any pet food purchased at the time of vaccination.
Monitor results	keep computer records of increased uptake.
Review plans	after the year to see how successful it was and what else can be done to encourage booster uptake.

Marketing is being handled increasingly well in many veterinary practices and its success depends on committed support staff understanding their marketing role and carrying it out with enthusiasm.

What support staff say

Q: Is sales a part of your job that you a) enjoy b) find easy or difficult to do?

Christine: 'I enjoy the selling and find it reasonably easy. I always ascertain the needs of the client. For example, for an elderly lady living on her own requiring a flea treatment for her cat, I would recommend a spot on product as it would be easier for her to use than a spray.'

Pat: 'Product sales are important to the practice, I enjoy this part of my job and find it easy. I try to sell on recommendation, i.e. a product I have used myself or one that other clients have recommended. I always explain the benefits of the service or the product I am selling.'

Liz: 'I enjoy advising clients on our services and getting them to buy associated products like food or pet toys.'

Elaine: 'I find selling our services is easy because I firmly believe in their quality. When a client says they have recently acquired a new puppy or kitten, I make a point of drawing their attention to the services that our practice nurses can provide, like new kitten/puppy advice, worming or flea treatment.

In the case of a new puppy, I tell them about the benefits of attending our six-week puppy course. In this way I usually manage to arrange an appointment with the vet for a first vaccination and, if possible, a nurse appointment on the same day, plus adding their name to the next puppy class.'

Margaret: 'I only really find it easy to sell products which I know and believe are good. I always tell a client if I actually use a product I am selling them, it's always good to sell on recommendation.'

Q: How are you involved in promoting and marketing your practice?

Pat: 'By being friendly and efficient, smart and well groomed.'

Elaine: 'Although I am not directly involved in sales as we have a pet shop, everyone in the practice is trying to find effective ways of improving/encouraging clients to use our services and our pet shop. Also departmental heads like myself have weekly discussions with each other and the practice manager to discuss new marketing ideas.'

Liz: 'I arrange client evenings and open days and promote our services by talking to clients.'

Summary

- Sales and marketing are very different processes but they are both essential for a profitable practice. A well-marketed practice will bond existing clients and attract more new clients, so providing more sales opportunities.
- Increased sales means increased profits, some of which can be re-invested in the practice in new and better marketing programmes, and so the marketing cycle is complete as shown in the figure below.

Figure 15 The marketing cycle

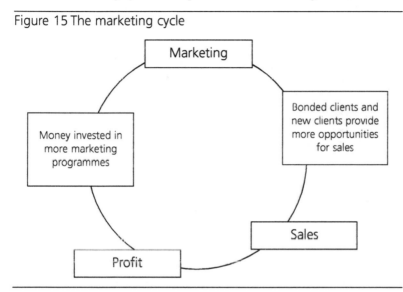

- Sales and marketing are very different processes – both essential for practice profitability – and support staff are involved in both.
- Selling is the promotion of veterinary services and products which results in the client making a purchase.
- Marketing is matching client needs and wants to the practice services in order to bond existing clients and sell more services to them and also to attract new clients.
- The main benefits of selling are increased profits and increased opportunities to bond clients.
- Support staff are the key figures involved in practice sales.
- Support staff should be aware of the difference between client needs and wants.
- Marketing is essential if a practice is to survive and prosper.
- Support staff are marketing to clients from the moment they walk through the surgery door to the moment they leave.

Exercise   7

List the ways you personally are able to market your practice internally to clients and externally to the local community.

8

Support staff and the law

'Veterinary practice is different from other businesses.' We have all heard this said and probably said it ourselves, but is it true?

Veterinary practice differs from many other businesses because it is a profession, but all professions – like the medical or legal professions, for example – have their own special problems, needs and peculiarities and in this veterinary practice is no different.

All practising veterinary surgeons must be members of the Royal College of Veterinary Surgeons (RCVS), the professional body which governs the conduct of veterinary surgeons. Membership of the RCVS gives vets the right to put MRCVS after their name, standing for Member of the RCVS. The powers of the RCVS are provided by the Veterinary Surgeons Act of 1966, the purpose of which is to

protect the public and animals from unqualified or inadequate practice and promote high standards of professional conduct.

There are statutory and ethical requirements set out by the RCVS to which all veterinary surgeons must adhere, and this of course affects how veterinary practices are run and the way support staff must carry out their roles. The RCVS rules pervade everything that the veterinary practice does. Businesses which are not professions (e.g. retailing), while subject to the law, are not regulated by statutory and ethical requirements to the same extent. This is the real difference between veterinary practices and other businesses. So how do the RCVS Regulations affect support staff?

Statutory requirements

The only people in a veterinary surgery who may treat ill animals are qualified vets who are members of the RCVS. Support staff must not diagnose or treat any illness in the animals brought to the surgery. The exceptions to this are qualified Veterinary Nurses (VNs) who, under

Schedule 3 of the Veterinary Surgeons Act, are allowed to carry out certain medical treatments and minor operations under the guidance, and at the discretion, of a veterinary surgeon.

The veterinary surgeon is accountable (legally responsible) for all the actions of their support staff and nurses. Should any incorrect treatment, diagnoses or advice be made by their support staff and nurses, it is the vet who the client may sue and who the RCVS may prevent from practising.

It is legally wrong, and enforceable by law, for a member of support staff to decide what is wrong with an animal and give the client advice on treatment. Support staff are often asked by clients to give advice: 'What do you think is wrong with Bonzo? Do you think he needs another course of those tablets he had last year or should I just worm him?' Although direct questions like this can be difficult the staff should always refer the client to the vet for advice: 'Well Mrs Jones, it could be a number of things, it's best to let the vet see Bonzo so that she can decide what should be done.'

Some clients will try to seek advice from support staff to avoid paying for a consultation but the support staff should never be tempted to give medical advice.

Trained staff can give general advice on worming, flea control, nutrition, weight control and so on, but if an animal is undergoing treatment a vet should also be consulted.

The vet is also responsible for the mistakes that staff may make. If the wrong tablets are dispensed or the wrong dosage or wormers given out, it is the vet who is answerable. The importance therefore of well-trained staff in a veterinary practice is obvious.

Veterinary surgeons do take out insurance to cover the possibility of mistakes both by themselves and other vets as well as by their support staff. The Veterinary Defence Society (VDS) is the 'insurance company' for the profession and deals with the claims made against veterinary surgeons by clients, as well as providing advice on how to handle client complaints and being sued. There were 700 claims made against veterinary practices in 1999. It has become more common to claim damages these days and sadly veterinary practice is no exception. Indeed, surprisingly, there are actually proportionately more claims against vets in the UK than in the USA.

Ethical requirements

On admission to the RCVS the veterinary surgeon promises to 'pursue the work of his profession with uprightness of conduct and that his constant endeavour will be to ensure the welfare of animals committed to his care.'

The RCVS produces a *Guide to Professional Conduct* containing the rules and regulations which vets must follow. The RCVS can remove veterinary surgeons from the Register if they contravene these rules by, for example, conducting themselves in an unacceptable way in relation to clients, staff or other vets. The *Guide* sets out the veterinary surgeon's obligations to the treatment of animals and the use of veterinary medicines and products, and their obligations towards clients and other veterinarians. These ethical obligations affect all the policies and procedures in the veterinary practice.

For example it would be convenient when Mr Brown, a notoriously bad payer, brings his dog for treatment to say, 'Sorry if you will not pay we will not treat your dog'. However, it is an obligation for all vets to relieve suffering, so Mr Brown's dog must be treated if it is in any kind of distress, even if the chances of payment are low. In cases of persistently slow payers and bad debtors the RCVS state that is acceptable to give the client notice in writing (by recorded delivery) that veterinary services will no longer be provided, and that the client must seek veterinary care elsewhere.

Confidentiality

One of the most important ethical requirements that affects support staff is confidentiality. Any information concerning an animal in the care of the practice is confidential and should never be divulged to a third party without the owner's consent, except in circumstances when the welfare of the animal is so at risk that it outweighs any obligation to the owner. Everyone likes to talk about their work, but staff must always be careful never to disclose information about client's pets.

The Data Protection Act 1998 is another way of ensuring client confidentiality. It protects the personal rights of clients whose private information is held on the practice computer or on client record cards. Businesses such as veterinary practices which hold personal details of clients would be wise to register with the Data Protection Registrar. Although recent correspondence in the *Veterinary Record* suggests that veterinary surgeries are not strictly required to register, as it depends on what the information is used for. The Data Protection Act sets out principles which all companies who have registered must follow. All client's details must be stored correctly and not be made available to outside bodies or kept longer than necessary.

Public liability

It is a legal requirement that all businesses must take out public liability insurance. The owner must ensure to the best of his ability that the public are not in danger or injured while on his premises, and should they be unfortunate enough to be so, then the business must have adequate insurance cover to pay for any claims for damages.

If Mr Green slips on the wet patch on the waiting room floor made by a previous client's dog (which the staff have not had time to clean up) and twists his ankle, he can sue the practice for injury. Having public liability ensures the claim can be paid without the business being affected.

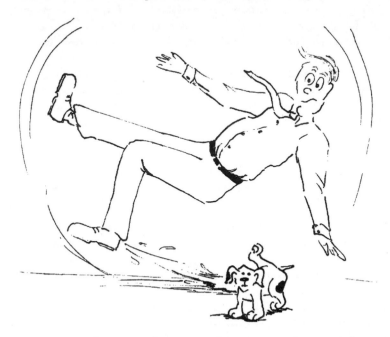

Ministry of Agriculture, Fisheries and Food (MAFF)

MAFF polices and enforces laws relating to animal health and welfare. They can impose movement restrictions on farm animals and appoint vets (called Local Veterinary Inspectors – LVIs) to oversee and enforce such restrictions. LVIs are also empowered by MAFF to supervise animal exports and the operation of slaughter houses. Small animal import and export is controlled by MAFF. One of the most recent pieces of legislation is the Pet Passport Scheme, allowing pets to travel to and return from specified countries without being subjected to quarantine regulations.

Employment legislation

Like all businesses, veterinary practices are subject to the ever-increasing amount of employment legislation which aims to protect employees from unfair dismissal and discrimination, and provides regulations for employee sickness, maternity, paternity and family leave. Most support staff will be aware of their employment rights, but if they have any queries they should consult the practice manager or the member of staff who is responsible for salary administration. If there are difficulties in finding out this information, it may also be advisable to seek information from an outside body such as the local Department of Social Security or Citizens Advice Bureau.

Health and Safety at Work Act

The Health and Safety at Work Act of 1974, and subsequent European and UK legislation, requires employers to ensure as far as is reasonably practicable the health and safety of their employees. It also requires employees to take reasonable care of their own and others' health and safety at work.

Like all other businesses, veterinary practices should have a health and safety policy and carry out risk assessments in the areas named in the regulations. Support staff should be constantly aware of health and safety matters in the practice and follow all health and safety procedures set down. (Chapter 6 deals with health and safety in more detail.)

Waste management and duty of care

All waste products must, by law, be disposed of in a safe and legal manner. The waste from a veterinary practice is divided into office waste, which is disposed of in the normal way by the local authority, and clinical and pharmaceutical waste which is produced as a result of the activities of the practice. Clinical waste is composed of tissue, swabs, blood, hair, sharps and whole bodies while pharmaceutical waste is all forms of medicinal waste. Both types are disposed of by special licensed waste carriers and must be stored correctly while on the veterinary practice premises.

Pharmacy regulations

There are strict regulations set out by the RCVS about the sale, supply, storage, record-keeping, packaging and labelling of medicines dispensed in veterinary practices. The BVA also produces a *Code of Practice on Medicines* which is issued automatically to all vets who are BVA members. The aim of the code is to provide guidance on best practice for prescribing and dispensing of medical products by veterinarians, and it also includes information and recommendations on drug storage, labelling, sale, supply, record-keeping and disposal.

Veterinary surgeons may only prescribe medicines to animals under their care and no one except the vet may supply medicinal products unless given authority by a veterinary surgeon.

Repeat prescriptions often cause support staff difficulty. The regulations states that for an animal to be given a repeat prescription, it must have been seen by the veterinary surgeon within a period of time set by the veterinary surgeon. This period of time is often in the region of six months.

When medicines are dispensed they must be labelled according to the labelling requirements of the RCVS. Labelling of medicines will be discussed in detail in Chapter 9.

Controlled drugs (usually Schedule 2 controlled drugs) must be kept in a locked medicine cabinet which can only be opened by the veterinary surgeon or a person authorised by the vet to do so. A record of all controlled drug purchases and dispensing must be kept by the veterinary practice.

Veterinary medicines must be prescribed using the cascade system which guides vets in the use of preferred drug treatment according to the product license the drugs have been granted. If a vet wishes to use a drug not named in the cascade he must be able to justify its use for the animal and the client must sign an agreement for its use.

The storage of drugs is a support staff responsibility and all drugs should be stored in accordance with the manufacturer's instructions and be protected from extremes of environmental conditions. The refrigerators in which drugs are stored should be temperature-monitored and recorded on a daily basis.

Returned drugs should not be reused, as their storage in the client's home may not have complied with storage regulations. Practices have different policies on returned drugs, but as a general rule, drugs may be returned for disposal but their cost not refunded to the client.

Welfare organisations

The best-known animal welfare organisation is the Royal Society for the Prevention of Cruelty to Animals (RSPCA). The RSPCA was the first animal welfare organisation in the world and the first law enforcement agency in the UK. During the first year of its existence in 1824, it achieved 149 convictions on charges of cruelty to animals. Although RSPCA personnel wear uniforms and are widely respected, they have limited powers. They do not have rights of entry and have to take police with them should entry to a property be required to rescue a distressed animal.

There are now many other animal welfare organisations, some of the better known being the Peoples Dispensary for Sick Animals (PDSA), National Canine Defence League (NCDL), Cats Protection League (CPL) and the Blue Cross. Veterinary contact with animal welfare organisations usually occurs when clients are referred to the organisations for assistance in paying veterinary fees, for help in re-homing their pet or if they are looking for a new pet.

The RSPCA may also call a vet to examine an animal which they suspect has been cruelly treated. This may involve treating the animal, observing recovery and gathering evidence for a prosecution. The vet may also be asked to act as an expert witness in court cases brought against individuals for potential cruelty. Should the animal belong to a client of the practice, this situation can give rise to a conflict of interest and many practices will not accept this role under these circumstances.

The selling of goods

Like most businesses the veterinary practice is subject to government regulations aimed at protecting the public. There is a lot of consumer rights law to protect clients against unfair trading and these are the three main ones affecting veterinary practices.

Sale and Supply of Goods Act 1994

A contract of sale of goods is a contract by which the seller transfers or agrees to transfer goods to the buyer at a price, as in the sale of dog food to a client.

Trades Descriptions Act 1968

A true and accurate description of goods or services must be given to a client; for example, how long a consultation lasts and what is included and not included in the price.

Consumer Protection Act 1987

This act protects consumers against defective goods and misleading price indications. For safety of the consumer, information must be given to clients on how to administer drugs to their animals at home to ensure their own safety.

Support staff should be aware of the implications of breaching these Acts and give true and accurate information about all goods and services the practice provides.

So veterinary practice differs from many other businesses in that it is governed by a professional body which regulates procedures and conduct. But in most other respects it is subject to many of the same legal requirements as any other business.

Support staff need to be aware of the ethical and statutory requirements applying to veterinary practice and how they affect their roles.

Summary

- All practising veterinary surgeons must be members of the R C V S.
- The R C V S sets *Guidelines* for professional conduct.
- Veterinary surgeons are accountable for the actions of their staff.
- Confidentiality must be maintained at all times.
- There is special legislation which applies to veterinary practices: waste management, pharmacy and M A F F regulations.
- Other important legislation which veterinary practices must comply with covers health and safety, employment and the selling of goods and services.

What support staff say

Q: What ethical matters have to be taken into consideration in veterinary practices that don't apply to other businesses?

Christine: 'The most important is client confidentiality.'

April: 'Confidentiality.'

Elaine: 'Due to the nature of the business it is highly unlikely that a vet will refuse to treat an animal, even if there is an outstanding account. It is because of this aspect that our accounts system has to be more flexible than other small businesses.

There have been one or two occasions when I have had to have a word with staff regarding confidentiality. Sometimes they have been talking about clients, unpaid accounts or specific animals – apparently completely oblivious, unconcerned that the clients in the waiting room could hear every word. I have explained that even if they are complaining about an in patient barking all day in the kennel, it gives a very unprofessional impression of the practice.'

Liz: 'The care of the client's animal is the most important issue and although we need the client to pay for treatment, we differ from other small businesses because of the animal care aspect.'

Margaret: 'Whilst vets must have good business management, they are also dealing with life and death and this does make a difference. Most vets would feel ethically bound to treat an animal even in cases of outstanding debt. I feel in the long run we are therefore bound to have more cases of outstanding debt.'

Exercise 8
Suggest four ways that confidentiality could be breached, including an example when using a computer. How does your practice safeguard against any breaches of confidentiality?

9

Support staff and the clinical role

Some veterinary practices have established defined roles for clinical and clerical staff, so that nurses are not involved with reception work and receptionists and administrators do not have any kind of clinical role. This is more common in large practices, as in small animal practices, with typically fewer employees, it is more difficult to have completely separate roles for staff and still be able to provide staff cover for holidays and sickness. Defined roles mean that staff become more specialised and expert in what they do, but it also means that they are less able to help in other areas of the practice if needed. The use of specialist or multi-skilled staff depends on the preference and organisation of the veterinary practice.

There are large numbers of support staff who are involved with clinical and nursing tasks, such as dispensing, helping the consulting vet and assisting at operations, as well as carrying out administrative and reception duties. Large numbers of nurses also take their turn helping at reception and doing a variety of clerical tasks, as well as nursing and caring for sick animals.

Consequently support staff require a sound knowledge of many of the clinical aspects of veterinary work.

Pet care advice

The veterinary practice may have specially trained staff running pet healthcare clinics, but it is still important that any staff who deal with clients can advise on basic pet care.

Staff should be familiar with:
- common breeds of cat, dog, rabbit, bird, fish, reptile and rodent
- common diseases of cats, dogs and rabbits
- common operations carried out on dogs, cats and rabbits
- oestrus cycles and gestation periods of the most common pets.

All reception staff should be able to give clients help and advice on basic animal care, such as how to choose a pet, feeding, housing, bedding, grooming and handling.

They should be able to give knowledgeable advice on vaccination and the benefits it gives. They should also be able to discuss flea and worm control with clients and give advice on the use of the different products available. Many clients require help on feeding their pets and all staff should be able to recommend suitable food for young, pregnant, old or sick animals, as well as those which simply require a maintenance diet or require a diet for a specific disease.

Staff will be able to refer clients to special in-house clinics for specific advice:

◆ puppy clinics
◆ adolescent clinics
◆ older pet clinics
◆ weight clinics
◆ dental clinics.

They still need to be able to give helpful general advice on all these pet areas because although not all clients will take up the opportunity of attending nurses clinics they still need to have basic pet care information.

Support staff working in reception will also need to talk to clients about exporting animals abroad and the pet passport scheme, which allows owners to take their animals abroad on holiday and bring them back without the need to place them in quarantine for 6 months. The advantages of pet insurance and microchipping are also important areas to discuss with clients.

Owners can insure their pets against injury and diseases, removing the worry of not being able to pay a large vet's bill if their cat or dog is involved in a RTA or develops a serious illness. Pet insurance, however, does not normally cover vaccination and routine neutering of dogs and cats. Microchipping involves inserting a very small microchip under the skin of the animal, usually at the back of the neck. This 'tag' has a unique number, and enables the lost animal to be identified by electronically reading the microchip underneath the skin using a microchip scanner. There is a central register of all micro-chipped animals so that, once the number has been checked, the pet can be identified and returned to its owner.

Support staff must be able to recognise animal emergencies and know the very basic first aid advice to give to clients if a vet is not immediately available. Here are some of the commonest emergencies.

Small animal

◆ anaphylaxis (severe allergic reactions, often from bee stings)

- bites
- poisoning
- cardiac failure
- heat stroke
- penetrating wounds of thorax or abdomen
- seizures.

Large animal

- bloat
- milk fever
- difficult calvings
- colic in horses.

Animal biology

It is a great advantage for the support staff who are not trained as VNs to have a basic understanding of the following areas which will affect their everyday work in the veterinary practice:

- anatomy and physiology
- parasitology
- microbiology.

Anatomy and physiology

Support staff spend a great deal of time talking to clients about their pet's health and welfare, the treatment and operations they may be having. It is of tremendous help if the staff understand a little of the biology of the cat and dog because it will help them to explain treatments and operations better and with more confidence. If they don't know what a dog's ovaries or uterus looks like, or where they are found in the body, it is much more difficult to talk with authority to the client whose most precious cat is coming in to be spayed tomorrow. How can you talk with confidence about dental procedures if you have no idea what a rabbit's teeth look like? Each day support staff book-in spays castrates, dentals, 'lump and bump' removals and so on. How many of these staff have actually seen these operations carried out? All support staff as part of their initial training would benefit from spending time in the operating theatre and the consulting room just to see and hear what goes on.

It is a great advantage if support staff are taught (the best way is likely to be at in-house training sessions) the fundamentals of:

- the cat, dog and rabbit skeleton
- teeth
- body tissues
- muscles
- body cavities

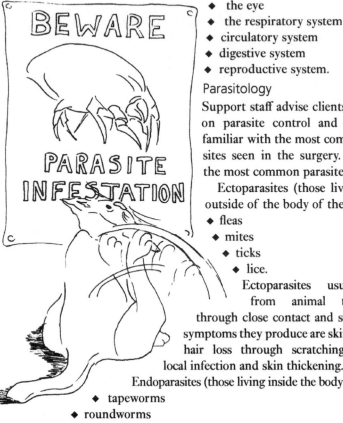

- the eye
- the respiratory system
- circulatory system
- digestive system
- reproductive system.

Parasitology

Support staff advise clients every day on parasite control and should be familiar with the most common parasites seen in the surgery. These are the most common parasites dealt.

Ectoparasites (those living on the outside of the body of the pet)

- fleas
- mites
- ticks
- lice.

Ectoparasites usually pass from animal to animal through close contact and some of the symptoms they produce are skin irritation, hair loss through scratching, anaemia, local infection and skin thickening.

Endoparasites (those living inside the body of the pet):

- tapeworms
- roundworms
- protozoa (parasites consisting of a single cell).

Most tapeworms and roundworms in their adult stage live in the gut of animals absorbing nutriments from the digesting food. Heavy infestations can cause severe loss of condition, dehydration and vomiting and diarrhoea. Roundworms can be anything from a few millimetres to several centimetres in length and consist of a muscular tube with a mouth and gut. Tapeworms consist of a head and a chain of segments, which may vary from two to three to a thousand; each segment contains eggs and when ripe is detached from the rest of the body and passed out in the faeces.

Many of these parasites can be transmitted from animals to humans (a process known as zoonosis).

The most familiar protozoan parasite is Toxoplasma, which can cause abortion in the cat and in sheep grazing on infected pasture. Toxoplasma is a potentially serious zoonosis for pregnant women, which may cause blindness or defects in unborn children. The actual risks from cats and dogs is low, and staff should be able to give sensible advice to clients who are worried about this disease.

Many ectoparasites, like the flea and most endoparasites, have complicated lifecycles with different stages of the life cycle living in different species of animal.

Microbiology

Micro-organisms cause a considerable proportion of diseases in clients' pets. Protozoans are the single celled organisms which cause such diseases as toxoplasmosis and coccidiosis. Bacteria cause diseases such as leptospirosis. Viruses cause feline leukaemia (F eLV), feline immunodeficiency (FIV), rabies, canine distemper, parvovirus, kennel cough and, in rabbits, myxomatosis.

Regular vaccination programmes can provide animals with immunity to these virus-borne diseases, and it is a support-staff role to explain the advantages and benefits of such programmes. As well as being aware of the different micro-organisms causing disease and the treatment, they should understand how immunity is provided by vaccination and why regular boosters must be given to maintain the pet's immunity.

Veterinary terminology

There are veterinary dictionaries which list the hundreds of veterinary terms which may be used. Staff responsible for typing reports or letters will benefit greatly from having a dictionary if only so that they are able to better decipher the veterinary surgeons' handwritten notes.

However it is important for staff to have a working knowledge of commonly used veterinary terms. A few common terms are given below, but staff would be advised to build up their own list as they come across the terms in practice or ask their veterinary surgeons for a list of terms they think staff should be familiar with.

Prefixes	meaning	*Example*	meaning
HYPER-	above	*hypertension*	increase in blood pressure
HYPO-	below	*hypoglycaemia*	low blood sugar
CYSTO-	bladder	*cystotomy*	opening of the bladder
HEPAT-	liver	*hepatosis*	liver inflammation
CARDIO-	heart	*cardiology*	the study of the heart
NEPHRO-	kidneys	*nephritis*	inflammation of the kidney
GASTRO-	stomach	*gastritis*	inflammation of the stomach
ENTERO-	intestinal	*enterotomy*	opening of the intestine
PYO-	pus	*pyometra*	pus in the womb
HAEM-	blood	*haematology*	study of blood
ENDO-	inside	*endoscope*	scope for looking inside cavities
ECTO-	outside	*ectoparasite*	parasite living on the outside of the host

Prefixes	meaning	*Example*	meaning
MYO-	muscle	*myocardium*	heart muscle
POLY-	excessive	*polymorphous*	many shaped
NASO-	nose	*nasolachrymal duct*	duct between nose and eye
OSTEO-	bone	*osteotome*	instrument for cutting bone

Suffixes:

-THERMIA	temperature	*hypothermia*	low temperature
-GLYCAEMIA	blood glucose	*hypoglycaemia*	low blood sugar
-ITIS	inflammation	*tonsilitis*	inflammation of the tonsils
-AEMIA	condition of the blood	*anaemia*	low blood cell count
-URIA	urine	*polyuria*	excessive production of urine
-DIPSIA	drinking	*polydipsia*	excessive thirst
-PHAGIA	eating	*dysphagia*	eating disorder
-ECTOMY	removal	*splenectomy*	removal of the spleen
-OTOMY	opening	*laparotomy*	opening of abdominal cavity

(incision into an organ, often for investigative purposes)

Other common terms are:

HAEMATOMA	blood clot
SEROMA	collection of serum
ECTROPION	eyelid turned outwards
ENTROPION	eyelid turned inwards
LAPOROTOMY	investigative surgery of the abdominal cavity
PRURITUS	itching
RENAL	kidney
ALOPECIA	hair loss
ERYTHEMA	redness of the skin

Veterinary assistance

Support staff may be called upon to assist the veterinary surgeon in the consulting room or the operating theatre, and to carry out laboratory tests and dispense medicines.

Consulting room assistance requires staff to be competent in animal handling, restraining and muzzling if required. They will need to be able to raise veins, help administer tablets and provide the vet with the medicines, materials, equipment and help they may need to carry out minor surgical procedures or examinations.

Support staff often have the responsibility of dispensing drugs to clients once the vet has examined the owner's animal. This is a very responsible role which requires considerable care and accuracy. Veterinary practices have their own dispensaries from which all drugs are dispensed. There are a number of different legal categories of medicines which veterinary practices dispense and all staff should be familiar with, and understand, the dispensing regulations for each:

Figure 16 The categories of medicines

GSL   **General Sales List**
Can be sold without restriction to anyone whether or not they are a client.

P   **Pharmacy**
May be supplied by vets for administration to animals under their care, or over the counter by a pharmacist.

PML   **Pharmacy and Merchants List**
May be supplied by a vet for administration to animals under their care or by a pharmacist or by a registered agricultural merchant.

POM   **Prescription Only Medicine**
May be supplied by vets for administration to animals under their care or by a pharmacist on a veterinary prescription.

CD   **Controlled Drugs, Schedules 1–5.**
Schedule 2 and 3 are the most common in veterinary practice. Schedule 2 drugs must be kept in a locked cabinet.

Staff responsible for drug ordering, receipt and storage should be aware of the need to follow manufacturer's instructions on drug storage and ensure drugs are kept at the correct temperature, away from light if instructions demand this, away from humid areas and flammable products and, for controlled drugs, in secure locked cupboards.

Dispensing drugs is a very responsible task. All drugs should be dispensed with care, checking that the correct drug and dosage is being dispensed. Each practice will have its own procedure for ensuring accuracy in dispensing procedures. All drugs must be labelled and the label must have the following information:

- client name and address
- animal name
- date
- name, strength, dose and quantity of drug
- veterinary practice name and address
- 'For animal treatment only'
- 'Keep out of the reach of children'
- withdrawal period (for food animal dispensing).

Pharmacy and dispensing is one of the most important areas concerning health and safety and here that the COSHH Regulations (Control of Substances Hazardous to Health) are most rigorous. Whenever they are dispensing, staff must always follow the practice standard operating procedures or rules on drug handling, as well as informing clients on the correct use of drugs which may present any kind of health and safety risk.

Assisting in the operating theatre is a specialist role and staff need to be well trained before they are asked to help veterinary surgeons with operations. They need to understand and be able to operate anaesthetic equipment, identify degrees of anaesthesia in animals on the operating table, be able to recognise the different surgical instruments and apply sterile and hygienic practice to all that they do.

Many veterinary practices now have in-house laboratories with staff carrying out biochemical and haematological tests and whole-blood profiles using electronic analysing equipment. Tests may be carried out on blood, serum and plasma, as well as skin scrapings for examination under the microscope. As well as being trained to test veterinary samples, staff must be very aware of safe laboratory practice, to avoid contamination and the spread of disease from infected material. In-house laboratory tests enable the vet to obtain quick results instead of having to wait for results from material sent to laboratories by post. There is an increasing trend to carry out in-house pre-anaesthetic blood tests which highlight any potential anaesthetic risks and allow the veterinary surgeon to use the most suitable anaesthetic for the animal. These trends will increase the laboratory work of support staff.

Veterinary hygiene

Good hygiene throughout the veterinary practice is very important to avoid the spread of disease, both to other animals and to staff. Cleanliness is important not only in the clinical areas but also in the waiting room which, as we discussed in Chapter 2, is the area of the practice that clients first see and which probably leaves the most lasting impression.

Staff should be aware of the correct use of disinfectants in the different areas of the practice, which disinfectant product to use, how often to clean floors, consulting tables, walls etc.

This is the least glamorous part of life in the practice but one of the most essential and no-one should be considered above taking their turn to wash, scrub or polish.

Waste disposal

Waste disposal is the other important aspect of veterinary hygiene. There are legal requirements which set down the ways of disposing of the type of waste produced in veterinary practices under the Duty of Care Regulations.

The table below shows the the types of waste materials produced by veterinary practices.

Figure 17 Types of practice waste

Office waste	- mainly paper and cardboard
Sharps	- needles, scalpel blades and small pieces of broken glass e.g. tops of vials
Clinical waste	- swabs, bandages, material contaminated by urine or faeces, body tissue, small body parts and euthanased animals
Pharmaceutical waste	- empty drugs bottles and syringes, out-of-date drugs and part used drugs.

General office waste is disposed of by local authority refuse collectors but all other waste must be collected and disposed of by registered waste disposal companies who have a current waste disposal license.

All staff should know the different categories of waste and how to dispose of them safely.

Summary

- Most veterinary support staff need to be multi-skilled and take on clinical as well as clerical roles.
- Staff should be able to advise clients on general pet care – healthy housing and feeding, vaccination, microchipping, taking animals abroad – and they must be able to recognise emergency situations.
- Support staff should have a basic understanding of cat, dog and rabbit anatomy and physiology, and be familiar with the common parasites and micro-organisms which cause diseases in pets.
- All staff should have a knowledge of common veterinary terminology.
- Support staff helping veterinary surgeons in the consulting room need to have good animal-handling abilities and be able to dispense medicines under the direction of the vet with care and accuracy.
- Those staff providing nursing assistance to veterinary surgeons should be trained in the use of anaesthetics and veterinary equipment.
- Veterinary hygiene and correct waste disposal is very important. All staff should be aware of correct hygiene procedures, the categories of veterinary waste and how it is disposed of from the practice.

What support staff say

Q: In what way are you involved with the clinical side of the practice?

Elaine: 'Mainly, I have to give advice to clients on flea and worming control. I attend the various drug and clinical treatment meetings we have in the practice, to keep up to date with new products and treatments.'

Margaret: 'Because I complete insurance forms I have to be familiar with new drugs, treatments and surgical procedures. I do this by attending training sessions held by the practice on new drugs etc. I often have to talk to the vets about an animal's treatment when filling in the insurance forms so I learn a great deal in this way as well.'

Liz: 'I oversee the running of the dispensary, this includes drug purchasing and being responsible for health and safety and COSHH. So I have to have a very thorough knowledge of all the drugs we use and how we use them, so that I can carry out risk assessments. I liaise with the drug companies and monitor discounts and special offers.'

Christine: 'I assist in the consulting room and operating theatre, I also clip nails, clean ears and de-matt animals coats. I advise on flea and worm control and nutrition.'

Exercise 9
Write down how you would advise a client on the purchase, care, housing and feeding of a new rabbit.

10

Teamwork –
Understanding other roles

For a veterinary practice to run efficiently and effectively, as well as profitably, all the staff must be working together towards the practice aims and objectives. Working well together is only possible if all the members of staff understand the practice's aims and objectives and also what the roles of the other members of staff are. Everyone needs to work as a team rather than as individuals who do not communicate with each other.

To work successfully with other members of the practice, support staff need to have a good understanding of the veterinary surgeons', nurses' and other support staff roles. This will enable them to understand and sympathise better with the difficulties other staff face in their daily routines. In the long term this understanding will result in much better teamwork amongst all the staff.

So often the problems which occur in practice are because of poor communication and a lack of understanding of each other's problems during the working day.

Understanding the practice aims and objectives

Aim – What are we trying to do?

Objective – How will we do it?

Support staff need to be sure of the practice aims and the objectives through which these aims will be reached. After all if they do not know the practice aims, how can staff be expected to work towards them or know what their jobs really entail?

Practice aims and objectives are usually listed in the practice manual, but if there is no manual support staff should make sure they ask the practice manager or a partner exactly what the aims of the practice are.

A typical practice aim would be:

To provide the best possible total healthcare for our clients' animals.

The objectives by which this may be achieved might be:
◆ preventative medicine
◆ surgical skills
◆ clinical treatment
◆ nurse's clinics
◆ modern equipment
◆ good client communication
◆ excellent client service
◆ client education
◆ high quality pet products.

Understanding your own role

Each member of staff should have a detailed job description listing all the tasks they are expected to carry out (full details of job descriptions are given in Chapter 11). All support staff should be absolutely clear what their role entails:
◆ Which tasks they carry out.
◆ Where they carry them out (main surgery, branch surgery).
◆ When they carry them out (full time, part time).
◆ How they carry them out (is there a receptionist's manual, for instance?)
◆ Who they are responsible to.
◆ Who they are responsible for.

The job description helps to avoid some of the misunderstandings which can so easily arise through a lack of understanding of one's own and others' roles.

Understanding the veterinary surgeon's role

Veterinary surgeons don't just see clients in the waiting room or carry out operations. They have many more roles as is shown below:
◆ consultations
◆ surgery
◆ home visits
◆ L / A visits
◆ night duty
◆ weekend duty
◆ telephone calls to client
◆ letters to clients
◆ talking to clients
◆ report writing
◆ Ministry of Agriculture work

- branch practice work
- attending training courses
- providing training for nurses
- working for a veterinary certificate
- practice meetings
- staff meetings
- departmental meetings
- practice administration
- thinking time.

Support staff do need to be aware of all these other roles and pressures on the veterinary surgeon's time. Then they understand why the vet is unhappy if, when Mrs Jones rings up to make an appointment for 10.30 and there is no available slot, because Mrs Jones will not accept alternative times and says her dog Popsie is ill, the receptionist 'slips in an extra appointment' before the 11.00 a.m. break, to keep Mrs Jones happy.

The receptionist is trying to provide a good service for the client and at the same time attempting to avoid the hassle she knows there will be if Mrs Jones does not get what she wants. But has she looked at the situation from the vet's point of view? Last night he was on duty and he was called out four times, with the last call at 3 a.m. So he's tired, still has to prepare for a dentistry course he is going on tomorrow, and in his mid-morning break he has six telephone calls to make to clients. He has already seen a series of rather awkward clients this morning and then just when he should be finishing, in comes Mrs Jones and she always has a hundred-and-one questions and overstays her appointment time.

It's easy to see why the vet is less than pleased with that appointment that was just 'popped in' and how these situations can lead to conflict. Consulting is a stressful business and the receptionist needs to have some sympathy with this. While, at the same time, the vet needs to be aware of the difficulties of running the reception desk and allocating appointments. It's all to do with understanding and communication.

When faced with the 'Mrs Jones' situation, the receptionist should be firm, offering Mrs Jones alternative appointments later in the morning, but not slotting her in at 10.55 a.m. By using the assertive techniques described in Chapter 4, the receptionist should be able to persuade Mrs Jones to accept the first available appointment convenient to the veterinary surgery and not give in to unreasonable demands. The conversation should go something like this:

> *I'm sorry Mrs Jones we simply do not have any spare appointments before 12.00. But I know the vet will really want to see Popsie, so can we book an appointment for her at 12.15 p.m? I'll explain to the vet how worried you are and I'm sure he will be able to help Popsie.*

Understanding the nurse's role

In larger practices nursing is often separated from other support staff roles and the many facets of the nurse's job are sometimes not fully understood by support staff. Nurses may take on any of the following roles:

◆ head nurse
◆ medical nurse
◆ surgical nurse
◆ hospital nurse
◆ practice nurse
◆ nursing clinics
◆ consulting nurse
◆ training other nurses
◆ training for their own VN qualification
◆ stock control
◆ dispensing
◆ x-raying
◆ lab work
◆ dental work
◆ animal nursing
◆ cleaning clinical areas
◆ client liaison
◆ client advice
◆ receptionist.

Like all support staff the nurses are usually trying to carry out a number of jobs all at once and if the other support staff do not appreciate these tasks, it will lead to difficulties.

Imagine: It's 8.30 a.m. on a busy Monday morning and clients are bring in their animals for the morning's operations. A queue has built up in the waiting room and some of the clients are beginning to get agitated in case they are late for work. Sarah and Jane the receptionists are trying to deal with these clients, as well as answer the telephone and see in the clients who have arrived early for their 9 a.m. appointments. The nurses who admit the animals for their operations seem to have disappeared. Finally Sarah telephones the prep room and demands that a nurse come up to the waiting room and 'sort out this mess'. This is not good for staff relations and both receptionists and nurses feel unjustly treated.

But has Sarah looked at the situation from the nurses' point of view? They are short-staffed in nursing that morning, the labrador which was admitted second became aggressive and it took two nurses to get it into a kennel. The hospital vet needed some help to treat a cat and an RTA was admitted. So Sarah's phone call was not appreciated.

There are two areas to consider here. It's true that the receptionists need to be aware of the different roles the nurses have and the process they go through when admitting an animal. But, at the same time, the nurses need to inform the receptionists that there is a hold-up in the admissions procedure. Once again it's all to do with understanding and communication.

Sarah should not have reacted as she did. She should have coped with the situation at the time and then arranged a time to talk to the nurse in charge of admissions, to both explain the problems they have in admitting animals and sort out what the best solutions will be. The situation comes back to teamwork, working together to solve difficulties, not against each other to create more problems such as, in this case, bad feelings and a poor image of the practice to the client.

Understanding other support staff roles

Support staff roles vary tremendously and can encompass any of the following activities:

◆ receptionist
◆ telephonist
◆ book-keeper
◆ client account manager
◆ secretary
◆ dispenser
◆ pet insurance administrator
◆ office administrator
◆ stock controller
◆ health and safety officer
◆ pet shop/sales manager
◆ animal care assistant.

Each of these roles involves many tasks and procedures and, just as with the two cases illustrated, a lack of understanding of, and empathy with, each others' roles can lead to conflict.

Teamwork and communication are the keys to solving much of the conflict caused by such misunderstandings.

Teamwork and communication

Teamwork

A team is a group of people working together towards a common goal. Teams require from their members:

Commitment – all members must believe in the work the team is doing.
Co-operation – all members must help each other and work together to achieve the overall goals.

Communication – all members must talk to each other about the work
  and any problems, difficulties or successes, at every opportunity.
Contribution – all members will have different roles and strengths but
  they must all pull their weight to contribute to the success of the team.
Individuals can achieve a great deal by working on their own but:

T – together
E – everyone
A – achieves
M – more.

The veterinary practice should be seen as one big team
consisting of all members of the staff who are working together to provide
a veterinary service for their clients.

Within this team are many smaller teams such as:

The Surgical Nursing Team providing the nursing support for the
  veterinary surgeons before during and after operations.
The Reception Team providing a reception service to clients.
The Veterinary Team providing the clinical expertise.
The Nursing Clinic Team providing a variety of health clinic services for
  clients' pets.
The Dispensing Team (mainly in larger practices) taking responsibility for
  the dispensary and stock control.
The Management Team – usually made up of practice manager and the
  partners – organising and managing the running and development of
  the practice.

The Admin. Team providing the secretarial, accounting and book-keeping services for the practice.

Figure 17   Teams in practice

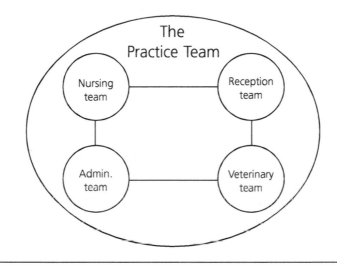

All these teams work as small units within the practice. The individuals in each team must communicate with each other, and the teams must communicate on a very regular basis with the other teams so that everyone is kept in touch with what is happening.

Some of the many advantages of teamwork are shown below:

➪ tasks can be carried out using everyone's skills.
➪ the members of the team are accountable to each other.
➪ teamwork provides and encourages the opportunity for communication and interaction with each other.
➪ team members can help each other, no one is left to work in isolation.
➪ teamwork helps to avoid misunderstandings and conflict.
➪ teamwork encourages feedback on ideas from colleagues.

Communication

Communication in the practice comes in many forms. It can be by:

Speaking – talking to other members of staff and giving them information.

Hearing/listening – to a member of staff giving information to others.

Writing – sending a memo or a message to other staff.

Reading – reading staff notice boards, newsletters and manuals

Seeing/observing – watching a demonstration, for instance, of how to deal with a difficult client in real time.

Communication with other members of the practice is essential and there are many ways this happens in the practice both formally and informally.

Formal communication

◆ One-to-one meetings – with supervisor, vet or practice manager, for a special reason or perhaps for an appraisal.
◆ Departmental meetings – perhaps the reception staff monthly meeting.
◆ Staff meetings – these may happen only once or twice a year.
◆ Team meetings – usually on a regular weekly or fortnightly basis.
◆ Practice manual – listing all the practice procedures and rules and regulations.
◆ Job manual – listing in detail the staff members' job tasks and how they are carried out.
◆ Practice internal newsletter – may be produced every month or more often, and contains information about new services, staff, products, procedures.
◆ Memos – sent to staff on specific topics which they need to know about.
◆ Notice boards – general information may be pinned to notice boards or there may be special notice boards for particular issues, such as health and safety.

Informal communication

◆ Talking to other members of staff during tea and coffee breaks.
◆ Talking to team mates whilst working.
◆ Managing to catch the occasional five minutes to talk to the vet.
◆ Social events – the annual barbecue, Christmas party or a night out bowling.

Communication will usually be a combination of some or all of the above methods; the important thing is that it happens and that everyone in the practice uses the system.

Summary

▪ All staff need to understand the aims and objectives of the veterinary practice.
▪ Staff need to understand each other's roles so that they avoid conflict.
▪ Teamwork and communication are the keys to solving many conflicts and misunderstandings.
▪ The veterinary practice is one big team working together with common aims.
▪ Within the big team are a number of specialist teams.
▪ Teamwork means that Together Everyone Achieves More.
▪ Communication can be in many different forms, the important thing is that everyone does it.

What support staff say

Q: How do you get everyone in the practice to understand each other's roles and work as a team?

Christine: 'I would not ask anyone else to do anything I would not do myself. Everyone should be encouraged to get involved in every aspect of the work and we should help each other as much as possible.'

Pat: 'By understanding the practice objectives, by being motivated and by all pulling in the same direction. Staff should feel appreciated but we should all accept advice and constructive criticism.'

Alison: 'By good management, by socialising together and by good communication.'

Sharon: 'By regular meetings, talking to heads of departments and by talking to each other.'

Elaine: 'I take a keen interest in the new services that become available in the practice and try to keep up to date with any changes in staff roles, so that I am aware to whom I should be directing enquiries. I attend the weekly small-animal staff meeting and the heads of department meetings so that I can pass on relevant information to the people in my department.'

Liz: 'It can be difficult, everyone needs to be aware of the aims of the practice and willing to work together rather than do their "own thing", oblivious to the needs of others. Communication is very important and if people feel they are part of the practice and valued then the teamwork will follow.'

Margaret: 'Morale should be kept as high as possible, the team needs a common aim and you have to foster team spirit by always providing a good example, and go the extra mile and help your colleagues. I think talking to people, helping them if I can, enables me to find out what problems they have in their job and it makes me understand their role better. It's all down to talking, communicating and caring about other people.'

Exercise   10

Pick a member of staff from your practice who does a different job to you and list all the duties you think they carry out, then ask them to do the same thing for your job. Swap the lists and discuss how accurate an idea you had of each other's job.

11

Surviving in veterinary practice

Whatever we do in life it helps to have some basic survival equipment to help weather the storms. A veterinary practice can be a great place to work, but there are a number of items of survival equipment, which help enormously to smooth the passage of the working day. It's possible to survive without them, but life is made much easier if support staff have at least some of the survival aids mentioned below.

Contract of employment

All employees must be given a written contract of employment by their employer within 13 weeks of their starting employment. The contract of employment is the statement of the main terms and conditions by which the employee is employed and is an essential document both for employee and employer. Employment contracts vary but all should give the following information and be signed and dated by the employer and employee:

- the employer's name
- the employee's name
- the date that the individual's employment began
- job title
- hours of work
- place of work
- salary
- overtime, if available or required, and overtime payment
- holiday entitlement
- sickness and sick pay
- pension arrangements
- benefits such as health schemes, bonuses etc.
- period of notice

- notes on disciplinary rules
- notes on grievance procedures and who the employee can apply to if they have a grievance.

A contract of employment cannot be altered by an employer without the consent of the employee, unless there are exceptionally good reasons which affect the running of the business.

Job description

It is absolutely essential that all employees have a job description. The job description describes in detail the tasks and responsibilities which comprise the job and which the employee has contracted to carry out. It sets out not just the responsibilities and tasks but also the limitations of the job, so that there are no misunderstandings between the employer and employee about what the job entails.

If an employee has no written job description, how do they know what their job is and how can they carry it out properly? Without a job description an employer cannot insist that an employee carry out a particular task if the employee feels it is not part of their job. At the same time however, if an employee does not have a job description it is difficult for them to refuse to carry out any task asked of them. Either way confusion and bad feelings are generated.

A job description should consist of:

- job title
- location of work
- hours of work and flexibility required
- the main purpose of the job – for example:
  To act as a veterinary receptionist providing information and advice and help to clients who come to or telephone the surgery.
- principal duties of the job – all the duties required of the job would be listed here
- reporting lines – who they report to and who reports to them.

A job description is likely to change as the practice develops new services, but any changes should be carefully discussed with employees before a new job description is produced.

Practice aims and objectives

All employees need to know what the aims and objectives of the practice are. In other words, what is the practice trying to do and how is it going to do it? (Aims and objectives are discussed in Chapter 10).

Practice aims and objectives are often stated in the practice manual or employee handbook, but anyone not sure of their practice aims and objectives should ask the principal or practice manager what they are.

The practice manual

This is sometimes referred to as the 'practice Bible' and contains all the essential information needed for a member of staff to carry out to carry out their job, following the correct practice policies and procedures. It also provides them with information about health and safety, discipline, grievances, codes of dress, security in the practice and much more. An employee will be given the manual when they first start work and it will also include their contract of employment and job description. The contents of a typical practice manual might be:

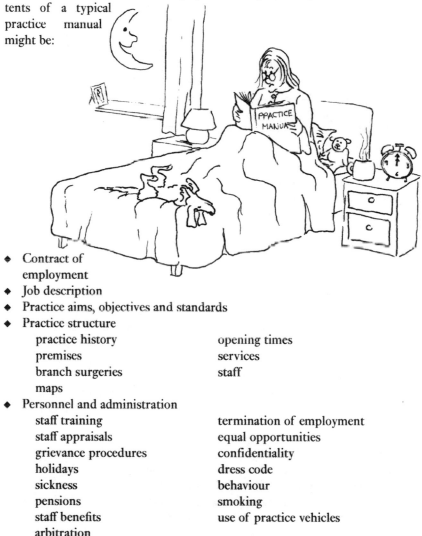

- ◆ Contract of employment
- ◆ Job description
- ◆ Practice aims, objectives and standards
- ◆ Practice structure

practice history	opening times
premises	services
branch surgeries	staff
maps	

- ◆ Personnel and administration

staff training	termination of employment
staff appraisals	equal opportunities
grievance procedures	confidentiality
holidays	dress code
sickness	behaviour
pensions	smoking
staff benefits	use of practice vehicles
arbitration	

- Health and safety
    practice policy
    fire safety
    duties of employees
    reporting accidents
- Client care and services
- Practice meetings
- Practice policies
- Standard operating procedures
- Local rules
- Security

The practice manual is an essential part of the survival kit but unfortunately not all veterinary practices provide one for their staff. Where a manual is not provided it is an excellent idea for employees to collect in their own 'manual' as much as possible of this essential information. Who knows, it may be that their personally compiled manual eventually forms the basis of an official manual for the practice.

The training manual

Many practices now have formalised support staff training programmes tailored to the needs of their staff and the practice. This organised training is in addition to the training that all staff will undergo when they first join the practice and learn how to carry out the tasks listed in their job description.

Whether staff benefit from a training programme, or are just simply sent on the occasional client care or supervisory skills course, it is definitely worthwhile to keep a personal training manual for the notes and details of all the training you have received. Details of flea-control products, wormers, vaccines, pet insurance, nutrition and all the other things clients may ask about can also be kept in the training manual, so that it can be referred to if in doubt. In time staff build up an excellent and indispensable reference tool to help them carry out their role in the practice.

Of course keeping a record of training is also useful, not only when staff have their annual appraisal, but also should they be applying for other jobs, as it can be used as part of their record of achievement in their job application.

Practice newsletters and information

It can be difficult to communicate in a veterinary practice and it sometimes takes a long time for information to filter through to all staff. Some practices produce internal newsletters, on a weekly or monthly basis, to keep staff informed of changes, new policies, new drugs and services. Others send out memos or have regular staff meetings and, sadly, a few don't seem to communicate at all! However these communications are worth keeping in whatever form they come, (make notes at staff meetings, if minutes are not circulated). File them in either the practice manual or training manual so that it is always possible to refer back to them if necessary.

The social side

This is a very good way to aid survival at work. It may be an organised staff meal or outing for all staff, or an impromptu get together of two or three receptionists, it doesn't really matter. A staff night out can release tensions and help individuals to get to know each other outside work. It's surprising how human even the most difficult staff members can become when they let their hair down a little and there aren't the constraints of work! These sort of social occasions help to bond employees and result in a happier and more supportive working environment.

The mentor

A mentor is someone who acts as a friend, guide and trusted counsellor to help and guide an individual through their life. This may be at work, at home, or during particularly difficult periods. They support and encourage their protegés to achieve their goals.

It can be a great aid to survival if a member of staff has such a person within or outside the veterinary practice. They will benefit greatly simply from having someone to talk to, discuss problems with and seek advice from. A mentor will support and encourage and it is always better to talk than to bottle up problems and emotions.

A sense of humour and a large jar of coffee

It could be argued that these two things are the most important items in the survival kit. Without a sense of humour no one goes far in veterinary practice and how could we get through the day without those endless cups of coffee?

Summary

- All employees should have a written contract of employment and job description.
- Employees should know the aims and objectives of the practice.
- A practice Manual gives employees information about the practice, the way it is run and the rules they must follow.
- A training manual gives employees information on how to do their job an should be added to as the job changes.
- Communication is vital to the survival of staff and the practice.
- Socialising with other colleagues and sharing common problems avoids some of the stress.
- No one survives without a sense of humour.

What support staff say

Q: What are the three most important things you need to survive in veterinary practice?

Christine: 'Patience, compassion and dedication but also a sense of humour, especially when it comes to registering some of the strangely named pets our clients have. Names such as Orgy, B******lugs and Darling are some of the ones which come to mind.'

Alison: 'A love of animals, patience and a sense of humour.'

Sharon: 'A sense of humour, compassion and you also need to understand your clients. Think of yourself as being one of them and treat them as you would wish to be treated.'

Pat: 'You need to keep calm and have a sense of humour. We have a client who always says, when he rings up to make an appointment, 'I want to make an appointment for the vet to see my crocodile'. (His pet is actually a cat). The first time he did this it was funny, the second time it was quite funny and after that it became tiresome, but we have to keep our sense of humour and patience.'

Liz: 'A sense of humour, a sense of humour and a sense of humour!'

Margaret: 'Stamina, being a team player and having a genuine desire to provide the best possible work you can do everyday.'

Elizabeth: 'A sense of humour, patience and understanding and a sound knowledge of your job.'

Elaine: 'It is essential to maintain a good sense of humour when working with over-stressed staff – whether they are vets, nurses or support staff. For example, there have been many occasions when it has been necessary for me to "chase" the vets to consult. If I had gone to them saying something like, "The waiting room is full, when are you coming to consult?" – the likelihood is that I would have been sent away with some terse comment. The trick is to know the people/personalities that you are dealing with and act accordingly. So saying "The clients will be breaking down the doors soon" or "We are knee deep in clients in the waiting room please come and save us" works wonders.'

Exercise   11

List your practice aims and objectives, then think of the activities you carry out in your job to achieve them e.g:

Aim – to provide a good telephone service to clients

Objectives – by...⇨ answering the phone within 3–5 rings
⇨ greeting the client ⇨ providing information ⇨ thanking them for calling
⇨ helping them to make appointments ⇨ saying goodbye

12

Support staff – the future

Changes in practice

The advent of corporate practice over the last few years has dramatically changed the traditional view of veterinary practices consisting of a main surgery and possibly one or two branch surgeries where all the staff know each other and the clients.

Corporate practice has resulted in multi-site practices often spread throughout the country with all sites displaying the corporate image both in design and management.

There has also been a significant increase in the number of practices with multiple premises or branch surgeries.

Practices generally are becoming larger although there are still a significant number of 'one man' practices. There is far more chance that in the future support staff will be working for a multi-site or larger practice, where they will need to communicate not only with staff at their own site but with colleagues at other sites and branches. The veterinary practice may not be quite the 'family' unit it once was. At the same time they are likely to benefit from a more highly organised management structure so that areas such as training, practice protocols and health and safety will be more formalised.

Practice organisation

The management of veterinary practices is continually improving which means that there is a corresponding improvement in personnel management. Contracts of employment, job descriptions, staff appraisals, health and safety implementation are just a few of the areas where support staff will benefit from this better organisation.

In order to carry out all these management tasks many practices now employ a practice manager who is responsible for managing the practice, finance, planning, marketing and health and safety as well as overseeing general practice administration. An important role for the manager is to forecast and plan for the future and, together with the partners, produce business plans looking at the services the practice will be providing in the future. If a practice does not have a practice manager they may have a practice administrator whose role is to ensure the smooth running of the practice admin areas. They undertake a variety of admin tasks including accounts, office administration, purchasing, insurance, rotas and IT. These administrative roles are increasing in veterinary practice and are ideal roles for some support staff to move into in the future, especially as formal training in practice administration is now available in the form of the Veterinary Practice Administration Certificate, which will be discussed later in the chapter.

As practices increase in size and specialise, so support staff roles also tend to become more specialist. This is seen particularly in nursing, where VNs may take on practice nurse roles, nurse management roles or specialise in, say, surgical nursing. The nursing role for other support staff is diminishing in many practices as they develop more structured nursing services and admin services. Many nurses are still involved with reception work but increasingly the traditional multi-skilled member of support staff is likely to be doing less and less nursing.

As practices increase in size and the numbers of support staff employed increases too, some support staff will have more supervisory roles and take on the challenge of leading teams of receptionists or office staff. Supervisory skills require people who will be able to organise teams, set rotas and holiday cover, handle discipline and take on personnel matters in their particular areas. Other roles may be responsible for client debt control, training new members of staff and carrying out staff appraisals for the people they supervise.

Government legislation will continue to increase, new health and safety and employment regulations alone have resulted in a large increase in administration time for veterinary practices and support staff are likely to play a greater part in helping to administer new regulations. Specialist admin roles for support staff are becoming more common. Practices may designate a particular member of support staff to implement their health and safety policy, deal with pet insurance claim forms, administer the practice website or run the practice dispensary and deal with stock control. Some members of support staff will need to be trained as the official practice first aiders, others may be appointed as fire officers or have specific responsibilities in health and safety areas.

Practice specialisation

Veterinary practices are becoming ever more specialised. There are specialist feline clinics and exotic clinics, and practices which concentrate only on alternative and holistic veterinary care.

Since the BSE and farming crisis a number of mixed practices have shed their large animal role and become totally small animal practices, and there are also an increasing number of referral practices.

The increase in specialisation requires a staff with more specialist knowledge and skills. This applies not only to the veterinary surgeons but also to the nurses and support staff who will be involved in dealing with clients who require specialist help and advice. The receptionist in an exotic's clinic will have an exciting range of reptilian and avian knowledge and identification skills, as well as being able to advise on general care of rabbits, hamsters and gerbils, the traditional alternative pets to cats and dogs.

The future will also see more support staff training as bereavement counsellors and behaviourists, nutritionists and pet insurance claim administrators. Nurses are also taking on more responsible roles in practice. There are now practice nurses and nurses who run their own nurse's clinics specialising in giving healthcare advice for puppies, adolescent or older dogs. Nurses also run weight and dental clinics and some specialise in behavioural advice. To carry out their support role the non-nursing staff will need to be fully aware of what these specialist nursing roles involve, so that they can talk knowledgeably to clients and advise them on the advantages of taking their pet to any of the clinics the nurses may offer. In addition to a good knowledge of the veterinary service being offered, good marketing skills will also be required here.

Night clinics are springing up in some of our cities involving a full veterinary service from 8.00 p.m. to 8.00 a.m. This will involve not only nurses but also other administrative staff in unsocial working hours.

Longer opening hours in line with those of the retail industry mean that all day Saturday and Sunday opening for veterinary surgeries will increasingly be expected and a seven day working week will be the norm for many staff.

Client expectations

Clients are becoming more informed and more demanding with much higher expectations of veterinary practices and their staff. The proliferation of veterinary TV programmes has made the general public far more familiar with veterinary medicine and has led to increased expectations for the treatment of their sick pets. Sadly these programmes do not inform the

public of the cost of veterinary treatment, especially for the more complicated and expensive procedures which are carried out. The public are
however generally better informed and support staff are increasingly likely to find that they will be asked more difficult and in-depth questions by
clients. This means that support staff may well need a greater degree of
understanding and knowledge in the future

'Pets as part of the family' is now a well used phrase and continues to be
an important aspect of client service for the veterinary profession. Pets are
more valued by their owners than they used to be. Not so very long ago a
cat or dog badly injured in an RTA would have probably been put to sleep
by the vet, an operation to repair the damage may not often have been considered by the owners. Today surgical techniques are constantly improving
and clients are willing to spend considerable amounts of money in order to
save the lives of their pets. Many pets are viewed as children or child
replacements. In a recent client survey which I carried out for a veterinary
practice, a client who was asked about the cost of veterinary fees replied
that she would spend anything to make sure her daughter received the best
medical treatment, and the same would go for their labrador as she was also
a member of family. House rabbits can cost their owners a considerable
amount just in vaccination, spaying or castrating and dental treatment, but
clients are quite ready to spend money on this furry friend.

Clients are also treating their pets as part of the family when it comes to
euthanasia. Many more clients request back the ashes of their pets after
cremation and the pet crematoria are flourishing, providing memorial
headstones for deceased 'loved ones'. An increasing number of clients use
bereavement counselling, provided by their veterinary practices to help
them get over the death of their pet. Support staff often play an important
role in bereavement counselling using the publications and courses provided by organisations such as The Society for Companion Animal
Studies to help them provide the correct counselling service to clients.

Clients are becoming more aware of alternative therapies in veterinary
practice and support staff in turn will need to be able to at least have
knowledge of these alternative procedures, even if the practice does not
provide them.

Sadly along with greater client expectations comes the increased tendency to sue the veterinary practice if something goes wrong. The
Veterinary Defence Society dealt with 700 claims against veterinary practices in 1999 and the number of advice calls has risen threefold since 1998.
Most of these claims are against veterinary surgeons but it is realistic to
expect that today any mistake however small may be the subject of a claim
against the practice.

Veterinary practices are likely in the future to be competing for a smaller market share of clients so the public relations and marketing skills of all the members of staff will be of even greater importance than at present.

The internet

It is estimated that 35% of the population now have access to the internet and that this will increase to 85% over the next five years. An increasing number of veterinary practices have developed their own websites, many of which have a client enquiry line. Support staff are going to be more involved in maintenance of websites as well as downloading and replying to client queries.

The many veterinary and pet product internet sites which have appeared over the last 18 months have meant that clients often come to the veterinary surgery armed with information about the diseases they think their pet has, and the treatments that it should have. The tact and diplomacy of the receptionist as well as the vet will be required more and more for these circumstances.

Websites only succeed if they are maintained and updated on a very regular basis. This is an excellent role. A computer literate member of the support staff is the ideal person to undertake this job. Website information will need to be continually changed and data put onto the site in areas such as:

◆ new staff
◆ new services
◆ practice news and events
◆ practice newsletter
◆ lost and found animals
◆ pet information
◆ special offers and promotions
◆ new products.

The proportion of clients looking at veterinary websites may be relatively small today but it may well increase rapidly over the next few years. Support staff will be in the forefront of fielding the increase in computer, internet and website work.

Competition

There has always been competition between veterinary practices but if current trends continue and the numbers of pets and clients decline this competition will become fiercer and the importance of bonding clients even more important. The Fort Dodge annual review for 1999 showed that active clients were down by 2%, new clients down by 17% and kittens down by 11% over the year and this trend continued into 2000.

Competition comes in the form of the large corporate practices whose economies of scale allow them to charge less for procedures and to open practices in areas where other veterinary surgeons might hesitate because of the competition from an existing practice.

Competition between neighbouring practices may well increase due to the decline in pets, loss of large animal work leading to more practices depending on the same small animal share of the market.

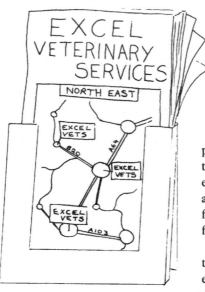

Pet superstores, especially those with veterinary clinics based inside, provide more competition in the form of not only pet product sales but also veterinary care.

Cheap vaccination clinics in some areas of the country also threaten local practices' income.

Internet sites offering cheap pet products may well encourage clients to buy on line rather than at the veterinary practice and free veterinary advice on line may prevent the client from seeking advice and treatment from their local vet.

The best way to beat the competition is to provide a service of excellence to the client. The people who play a major role in this are the support staff – the first and last point of contact with the practice for a client. It will be their role to provide a quality service, help to bond clients and exceed client expectations.

Good sales and marketing techniques will play an increasingly important part in bonding clients to the practice. More and more support staff will be at the cutting edge of marketing initiatives to bond existing clients and attract new ones. Sales of pet foods and products will continue to help finance the practice and it is important that support staff are better trained in sales techniques.

Practice public relations will also have to improve and many more practices may be using the media to market their services. Support staff will become involved in this area, be it posing behind the reception desk for a photo in a local newspaper or talking to clients at a practice Open Day. There may even be the occasional TV appearance – all part and parcel of the support staff role!

Training

To provide a quality service, staff need to have quality training. Staff training programmes are being developed in an increasing number of practices. Formal training for support staff has been somewhat neglected due in part to the lack of appropriate courses. Staff training programmes look at the needs of the practice and the individual and are tailor-made to improve the development of the employee. Such programmes are delivered as a mixture of in-house training, external courses and self-development and work well in the practices which run them. Many other kinds of training methods are likely to be used to train staff, below are just a sample of the training now available:

- in-house training by vets, nurses and administrative staff
- in-house induction courses
- books
- CD Roms
- internet training courses
- veterinary company sales and marketing meetings
- veterinary company product training courses
- external courses provided by veterinary companies, such as Hills
- external courses provided by independent veterinary trainers
- external non-veterinary administrative and management courses
- Veterinary Practice Management Association courses such as the VPAC
- Veterinary Practice Management Association regional meetings and conferences
- veterinary association meetings and conferences.

A few words about the Veterinary Practice Administration Certificate (VPAC) designed and offered by the Veterinary Practice Management Association (VPMA). This will provide the type of support staff training which has been lacking and will help support staff to improve their administrative skills, develop their roles within the practice and allow them to move into practice administration. The course, which will be delivered initially by agricultural and nurse training colleges, starts in 2001 and will cover:

- office procedures
- finance
- information technology
- marketing
- personnel
- ethics and statutory requirements
- customer care
- basic veterinary support.

The course is nationally accredited which means that the qualifications gained (all of which are assessed, not examined), will be recognised as achievements outside as well as inside the veterinary profession. This means they can be taken with staff who move on to other jobs and careers as proof of academic studies and qualifications.

There is also a role for some support staff in staff training, in particular for senior receptionists and nurses who will be increasingly involved in the initial in-house training of new employees. This sort of training has always taken place but on a fairly limited and informal basis. As practices develop more formal training programmes, staff training will take on more importance and more time will hopefully be devoted to it, giving staff trainers the time to plan and prepare for training sessions.

The privilege to dispense

Dispensing medicines to clients is a very responsible task which is carried out by both nurses and support staff in most practices. As practices increase in size there is a greater tendency to have dedicated dispensers running a practice dispensary. All medicines and repeat prescriptions are dispensed by the dispenser and no other staff are involved. Turning dispensing into such a specialist role enables the staff involved to have a high degree of familiarity with all the drugs and they can talk to the client with more knowledge. Dispensing staff will usually also be responsible for drug ordering and stock control. As practices enlarge there may well be an increasing need for this specialist role, however there is at the moment a rather large cloud on the horizon.

The veterinary surgeon has a privilege given to him by the government to dispense drugs; Parliament is considering removing this privilege. High street pharmacists instead of veterinary surgeons would then carry out dispensing of animal medicines.

At the time of writing, this issue had not been resolved but if veterinary surgeons lose this privilege the effect on veterinary practices and support staff could be significant.

If a practice cannot dispense then it does not need dispensers and it does not need anyone to organise drug ordering or stock control and there will be no repeat prescriptions to put up. This means fewer staff will be needed.

The future

The future is bright, but it will mean changes and challenges for veterinary support staff. This often untapped resource of skilled and committed people will be used much better by their veterinary practices. In the future support staff will take on more responsibility for the administration of the practice and will be helped to carry out their job better through improved training. 'Sitting by Nellie' to learn the job will still be part of the training, but only part, as practice training programmes are developed to address the training needs and development of all the practice staff.

So support staff in the future will be better trained and encouraged to develop new skills in the veterinary practice to enable them to provide the service that clients now expect. As nurses also become more highly trained and specialised so it is likely that other support staff will carry out fewer nursing roles.

Through support staff administration courses like the VPAC, staff will gain a greater awareness of the business of veterinary practice, how it is managed, and external and internal influences on its survival and financial success.

Summary

- Support staff are likely to specialise more in particular areas, such as health and safety, pet insurance, behaviour, bereavement counselling, marketing, nutrition counselling and supervisory skills.
- There will still be the routine jobs and the nasty jobs that all staff have to cope with in veterinary practice but support staff will also have a more interesting, challenging and participative role in veterinary practice.
- Corporate practices are likely to increase in number and smaller veterinary practices increase in size.
- Veterinary practices are likely to become more specialised, requiring staff to have greater specialist knowledge.
- Client expectations will continually increase. They will be willing to spend money on the pets they consider part of their family but they will also be more likely to make insurance claims against practices for negligence.
- The internet will have an increasing impact on veterinary practices and more practices will have their own websites.
- Competition will increase, mainly because there is a declining client/pet base but it will also come from larger multi-site practices.
- Support staff training will be more available and many practices will provide better training for their staff.
- Support staff will need to develop new and more specialised skills to continue to provide excellence in client service.

What support staff say

Q: How do you see your job changing in the future?

Pat: 'I think it will be more demanding. I will have more access to training to help further my skills.'

Alison: 'Promotion.'

Sharon: 'I will be doing more accounting and more invoice processing.'

Sheila: 'I will be assisting the practice manager and carrying out more admin.'

Elaine: 'The practice will need to constantly improve customer service and cash flow and my aim will be to ensure this happens.'

Liz: 'I think I will be taking on more management responsibilities.'

Margaret: 'I would like to be involved in helping to increase the uptake of pet insurance and help to organise the promotion of new services, such as our acupuncture service.'

Elizabeth: 'I think my job will become more computerised.'

Exercise   12

How do you think your job may change in the next five years?
List the areas of your job you would like to develop and any other roles you would like to carry out in the practice. Take the opportunity to talk to your practice manager or managing partner about how you would like to develop your role in the practice.

The last word from the support staff

What I like most about my job:
> working with people
> the variety
> no two days are the same
> meeting new challenges
> the times when I do some nursing
> dealing with clients and animals
> the variety of different jobs
> working independently
> the people I work with.

What I like least about my job:
> even though you try your best, you cannot please everyone
> having to carry out health and safety assessments
> being asked to do too many things all at once
> trying to sort out computer problems
> filling up the dog food stand
> running out of time
> all the extra paperwork we now seem to have
> poor staff communication
> temperamental vets
> when the phones won't stop ringing (all four lines at once)
> folding booster reminders.

The one thing I would like to change about my job would be:
> more nursing
> nothing (four support staff said this)
> more space to store things
> to have one day helping the nurses
> to have some holiday cover
> to stop checking and filing lab reports
> to have a more defined role, being so flexible can lead to you being over-stretched
> the phone system, so that I am not interrupted so much.

Glossary

BSAVA	British Small Animal Veterinary Association
BSE	Bovine Spongiform Encephalopothy
BVA	British Veterinary Association
BVNA	British Veterinary Nursing Association
CD	Controlled Drug
COSHH	Control of Substances Hazardous to Health
CPL	Cats Protection League
GSL	General Sales List
L/A	Large Animal
LVI	Local Veterinary Inspector
MAFF	Ministry of Agriculture, Fisheries and Food
MRCVS	Member of the Royal College of Veterinary Surgeons
NCDL	National Canine Defence League
NI	National Insurance
P	Pharmacy
PC	Personal Computer
PDSA	Peoples Dispensary for Sick Animals
PAYE	Pay As You Earn
PML	Pharmacy and Merchants List
POM	Prescription-only Medicine
RTA	Road Traffic Accident
RCVS	Royal College of Veterinary Surgeons
RSPCA	Royal Society for the Prevention of Cruelty to Animals
RIDDOR	Reporting of Injuries, Diseases and Dangerous Occurrences Regulations
S/A	Small Animal
SMP	Statutory Maternity Pay
SOP	Standard Operating Procedure
SSP	Statutory Sick Pay
VAT	Value Added Tax
VDS	Veterinary Defence Society
VN	Veterinary Nurse
VPAC	Veterinary Practice Administration Certificate
VPMA	Veterinary Practice Management Association

Index

Useful addresses

British Small Animal Veterinary Association
Woodrow House
1 Telford Way
Waterwells Business Park
Quedgeley
Gloucestershire G L 2 4BA
Tel: 01452 726700
website: www.bsava.co
email: adminoff@bsava.com

British Veterinary Association
7 Mansfield Street
London W1M 0AT
Tel: 0207 636 6541
website: www.bva.co.uk

British Veterinary Nursing Association
Level 15 Terminus House
Terminus Street
Harlow, Essex CM20 1XA
Tel: 01279 450567
email: bvna@compuserve.com

HSE Books
PO Box 1999
Sudbury
Suffolk CO10 6FS
Tel: 01787 881165

Health and Safety Executive
Information Centre
Broad Lane
Sheffield S3 7HQ
Tel: 0541 545500
www.open.gov.uk./hse/hsehome.htm

Royal College of Veterinary Surgeons
Belgravia House
62–64 Horseferry Road
London SW1P 2AF
Tel: 0207 222 2001
email: admin@rcvs.org.uk
website: www.rcvs.org.uk/rcvs/

Veterinary Practice Management
  Association
60 Stanley Street
Rothwell
Kettering
Northants NN14 6EB
Tel: 07000 782324
email: vpma@adminsupport.demon.co.uk
website: www.vetsonline.com/vpma